A YOUNG PERSON'S
GUIDE TO LIFE AND LOVE

A Young Person's Guide to Life and Love

Dr BENJAMIN SPOCK

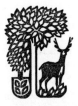

THE BODLEY HEAD
LONDON   SYDNEY
TORONTO

ISBN 0 370 01565 7
© 1970 by John D. Houston II, Trustee
Printed in Great Britain for

The Bodley Head Ltd

9 Bow Street, London, WC2E 7AL
by Richard Clay (The Chaucer Press), Ltd
Bungay, Suffolk
Set in Linotype Plantin
First published by Simon and Schuster, New York, 1970
This edition first published in Great Britain 1971

AUTHOR'S NOTE

For their advice and help in the preparation of this British edition of my book, I would like to thank Dr Julia Dawkins and Mr O. J. E. Pullen, formerly H.M.I., Staff Inspector for Health Education at the Department of Education and Science.

CONTENTS

I. How Man Gets His Nature

Attitudes towards Sexuality, 12
The Three-year-old Overestimates his Parents, 14
Romantic Love of Parent, 17
How Ideals are Set, 18
Attachments must be Broken, 19
Interest in God, Science and the Three R's, 21
Puberty and Adolescence, 22
How Humans Get their Attitudes towards Sex, 25
Why is Sex often Considered Sinful?, 28
The Question of Sexual Freedom, 30
The Relationship between Educational Level and
    Sexual Inhibition, 33
Contrasts in Sexual Behaviour in Boys and Girls, 35
Rivalry with Parents and the Search for Identity, 39
The Meaning of Marriage, 47
Patterns of Lovemaking, 52
Temperamental Differences between the Sexes, 55
Rivalry between the Sexes, 60
Occupations for Women and Men, 65

II. Boy–Girl Relations in the Teens

The Contrast between Romantic Love and
    Physical Sex, 72
Early Dating and Going Steady, 76
Dehumanisation of Love in America, 77
Illegitimate Pregnancy, 78
The Question of Petting, 81

Group Companionship, 87

Romance and Sex in Later Adolescence, 90

'The Arrangement' (Young People Living
Together without Marriage), 92

Falling Out of Love or Being Jilted, 94

To Tell or not to Tell, 97

Shyness is not a Bad Sign, 99

How to be Popular, 100

Dress, 104

III. LOVE, PSEUDO-LOVE AND SEXUAL DEVIATIONS

Varieties of Love, 110

Emotions Masquerading as Love, 111

Attraction only to 'Bad' Girls, 113

The Lechery of Males, 114

Scalp Collectors, 115

Possessiveness and Jealousy, 115

Sexual Deviations, 116

Homosexuality, 117

Sadism and Masochism, 121

Some other Deviations, 123

Obscenity, 125

IV. ADOLESCENT WORRIES

Self-consciousness and Fear of Illness, 130

Masturbation, 130

Ache in the Groin, 132

Impotence, 133

Frigidity, 135

CONTENTS

V. Anatomy and Physiology of Sex

Prepuberty Growth Spurt, 138
The External Genitals, 141
The Internal Genitals, 144
Menstrual Periods, 147
Nocturnal Emissions, 148
Contraception, 148
Abortion, 151

VI. Physical Conditions

Venereal Diseases, 154
Acne, 158
Body Odour, 160
Hair and Scalp, 160
General Health Care, 161

VII. Smoking, Alcohol and Drugs

Tobacco, 164
Alcohol, 165
Marijuana, 167

VIII. Delinquency

Conscience and Punishment, 170

IX. Relations with Parents

Gaining their Confidence, 176
Blaming Parents, 179
Sex Education, 182

9

CONTENTS

X. AFTERWORD

The Future, 186

Suggested Books for Further Reading, 189
Index, 190

[I]
How Man
Gets His Nature

Attitudes towards Sexuality

A fifteen-year-old girl said to me, 'Most of my friends have decided that sex is just a matter of glands.' This jolted me. I didn't think it was true. Still, I could understand why a young person could come to such a conclusion, in this mixed-up twentieth century. One problem is that sex seems to have entirely different meanings to you at different times, and also to different people. It can be a yearning to take tender care of your beloved. Another day it is a daydream about some physical intimacy, perhaps with a person you don't respect, which seems shocking. You may hear a strict priest or minister quoted as saying that sex is a sin except when it is used for the purpose of having children, or that even sexual thoughts are sinful. Another clergyman says that God made sex to be enjoyed. Lots of jokes and stories imply that sex is more pleasurable when it is illegal. Parents talk at different times as if sex were an exalted form of love or a dangerous trap or a joke to snigger at. Teenagers often decide that adults are hypocrites.

Teenagers often complain that the explanation of sex in books and lectures, or even in a frank talk with an older friend, leaves them feeling still in the dark, cheated. They are right. Sex isn't just a matter of how men's and women's bodies are shaped (anatomy) or how their bodies function (physiology) or how they are attracted towards each other (psychology). You gradually come to realise that sexuality in the broadest sense is an incredibly complex mixture of intense feelings not only towards other persons but towards beauty of all kinds and even towards your own aspirations

12

for your life. It can't be described adequately by words or diagrams any more than music can. Even the sexual experiences that a teenager may have in dating or dreaming will leave his understanding incomplete until he has grown up and has formed a deeply loving, permanent relationship.

The most important job I have to do in this book—and I'll start right away—is to explain how different sex and love are in a human being from what they are in other animals. To make this clear, I have to describe the complicated development of a human's feelings, beginning in infancy, and compare them, for example, with the emotional development of a puppy.

Some of these explanations of what goes on in the unconscious layers of the mind in childhood will sound unlikely and morbid to you. I would much prefer not to get into the matter of the unconscious, to keep things simple. But the problem is that I'm trying to explain why attitudes towards sexuality on the part of adults and young people and deviant people are so often baffling, contradictory and even weird-seeming. I'm also trying to explain the relationship of human idealism, creativity and spirituality to the inhibition and sublimation (modification) of sexuality in childhood. These are two central purposes of this book and I can't accomplish them without getting into the unconscious.

In earlier centuries there was no knowledge of the unconscious (because Freud hadn't unearthed it), but young people were not demanding a rational explanation of sexuality either. Sexuality, to the extent that it was dealt with officially in Western countries, was dealt with by religion. Religion said sex was predominantly dangerous and wicked except as it was justified in the creation of children. So youths had to worry about it, and enjoy it as far as their consciences allowed, but not raise questions, which might only serve to incriminate them.

13

The Three-year-old
Overestimates his Parents

A puppy goes through a brief dependent infancy in which his mother nurses him, guards him, teaches him about toileting and hunting. Then he becomes progressively more independent of his mother and she loses interest in coddling him any longer. Before long he is sexually mature. A male will be drawn to any female who is on heat without much discrimination. And every time a female is on heat (when her uterus is ready to grow a litter of puppies and she feels emotionally responsive to sexual relations) she will be receptive to a variety of dogs, whether she knows them or not. She will be receptive to her brother, father or son, if they happen to be around. In other words, sex for dogs is a matter of glands rather than of a very special attachment. But even in animals, sex is partly dependent on deep psychological factors. Experiments with monkeys, for instance, have shown that if from birth an infant is kept strictly isolated in a cage, away from any contact with his parents or others, he will have no desire for a sexual act when he is grown up and cannot be easily taught to try it.

The childhood of a human being is infinitely more complex. He is helplessly dependent on his mother for his whole first year. He spends the next two years insisting on his right to be a little more independent, exploring his small world and doing simple things for himself. (He can be quite obstinate and cranky about his rights.)

Then in the three- to six-year-old period he turns back more positively towards his parents. He comes to admire and love them extravagantly. He thinks they are the most wonderful, powerful, wise, attractive people in the world. He wants to be as much like them as he can, to learn to do

14

everything they do. This is Nature's way of civilising him, shaping him, inspiring him, for adulthood.

A boy now realises that it will be his destiny to grow up to be a man, and this makes him much more keen about copying the masculine activities of his father and other friendly men. (Back when he was two, he'd just as soon play with dolls.) Now he pushes toy cars and trucks around the floor. He pretends he is driving an imaginary car and makes the same kind of remarks that his father does. If he plays house with other small children, he wants to be the father of the family. He pretends to go to work after breakfast, to come home for supper. He carries on a solemn conversation with his 'wife' and scolds the children. This process goes way beyond simple imitation of acts. The boy is preparing himself for manhood—in attitude, in ambition, in spirit. We see this proved negatively in the rare case of the boy who, because of unusual influences, models himself after his mother instead of his father and never acquires masculine interests or a masculine manner.

A little girl between three and six realises she is going to be a woman some day, so she tries with particular delight to be like her mother, whom she considers to be the most beautiful, well-dressed, smart, rich woman in the world. She wants to do housework. She tries to take care of her dolls the way her mother cares for the baby. If she plays house she prefers to be the mother. She likes to dress up in her mother's clothes, and walks and talks just like her. When a four-year-old girl scolds her doll she sounds exactly like her mother. In spirit she is already a woman.

In the three- to six-year-old period boys as well as girls become intensely interested in where babies come from and how they are made. Girls are delighted to hear that they will grow babies inside themselves some day. This will be one of their deepest satisfactions in life—first in anticipation, later in reality, finally in retrospect. It's not as commonly known that boys at three and four years want to be able to do the same thing. This wish is so strong that when their mothers tell them it's impossible they often refuse to believe it. 'I can if I want to!' they say with vehemence. We believe that this envy of girls goes deep in all boys, even though they may not be conscious of it, and is an important element in their compensatory drive to be creative in other ways—to invent things, to build things, to write literature and music, to paint pictures, to make scientific discoveries. In most parts of the world older boys and men are ashamed, as a result of their upbringing, to admit they would like to grow babies. But in a few places, when a woman goes into labour and is taken to a special building to be attended by other women while she is giving birth, her husband complains of labour pains, too; his men-friends take him to the building reserved for men in labour and they comfort him while he writhes and groans. This sounds ridiculous to us, but they take it very seriously. I bring it up because it helps to explain the restless creativity of so many boys and men.

Another development still at approximately three years of age is that boys and girls usually misinterpret the meaning of their physical sexual differences. Psychoanalytic studies show that instead of realising that they are meant to be that way, they both jump to the anxious conclusion that a girl as well as a boy is meant to have a penis and that something unfortunate has happened. The girl usually decides that her mother didn't love her well enough to make her right or allowed some injury to occur; this disturbs her and makes her resentful of her mother and have feelings of rivalry towards boys. The boy decides that if an injury could happen to her it could happen to him, and this makes him somewhat anxious about his genitals and about his masculinity, consciously or unconsciously, all his life.

If parents try to discourage their small children from touching their genitals by implying that this might cause some kind of injury, as a majority of parents do, this naturally reinforces the anxiety about the genital differences.

Romantic Love of Parent

In the three- to six-year-old period a boy acquires a new attitude towards his mother. Previously he loved her in an infantile dependent way because it was mainly she who fed him and comforted him. But now that he is trying to grow up to be a man like his father, he becomes more and more romantic in his feelings for her. He begins to love her as a member of the opposite sex. He feels that she is the most fascinating female in the world. By the time he is about four years old he may say that he's going to marry her some day. This sounds silly to older children and adults. But to the little boy who doesn't yet realise that people marry only those their own age, it's a natural thing to love most the woman who has been a hundred times more important to him than any other woman or girl.

The boy at three and four becomes a romantic male not only because he wants to be like his father but also because his glands are beginning to turn his thoughts and feelings towards sex to a mild degree—though not nearly as strongly as in adolescence and adulthood. A little boy easily gets involved in sex play at this age and wants to see other children undressed. He may suggest to a girl friend that they undress and look at each other's bodies. This is a great age for playing doctor because that game gives an excuse to undress and look and touch. A boy is apt to lean against adults of whom he's fond and to touch his own penis for pleasure.

17

In a similar way a little girl at three and four will fall in love with her father, whom she now considers the most attractive and powerful man in the world. She develops this feeling partly because of wanting to be like her mother and also because her glands are beginning to influence her emotions. She also easily gets into sex play with others or herself.

How Ideals are Set

So the young child sets his own aspirations for life very high by greatly overestimating the magnificence of the parent of the same sex and resolving to grow up to be just like him. And, by overestimating the attractive qualities of the parent of the opposite sex, he forms his romantic* ideal.

What sort of person a boy's mother is, what her attitudes are to him and to her husband, will have a strong influence on the kind of girl he will later love and marry (quiet or jolly, for instance, assertive or agreeable, modest or exhibitionistic) and on the relationship they will have together. A girl's romantic ideal is formed by her image of her father. I don't mean, though, that a young man looks for an exact replica of his mother or a girl for a copy of her father—they may even be searching for certain characteristics that are quite opposite to those of their parents.

* From here on I will have to use the term 'romantic love' to mean a love for a person of the opposite sex which is spiritual, tender, and idealistic as well as physical. 'Romantic' is not a satisfactory adjective in the twentieth century because it is often used to indicate a sentimental, immature attitude. For instance, the phrase 'a romantic young girl' usually means a slightly silly one who is more in love with love than with a real person. But the alternative words are less satisfactory. The adjective 'sexual' by itself means to many people only a physical attraction. And it's too clumsy to say 'physical and spiritual' in every sentence.

Attachments must be Broken

But it wouldn't do if a boy remained tied romantically to his mother for life, or a girl to her father. They'd never get interested in other members of the opposite sex and they'd never want to leave home. Several factors work together to break up the attachment, and to discourage interest in sex generally, beginning at about five years of age. Freud, in his exploration of the hidden levels of the mind, found that feelings of rivalry towards the parent of the same sex—and a certain awe and fear of that parent—are the main cause of the suppression.

When a person loves another romantically, he's likely to become jealous if he finds he has a serious rival. The little boy, by about five years of age, is getting old enough to realise that he can't have his mother to himself because his father and she love each other and are very much married already. This upsets him in several ways. It discourages him. It makes him, in his hidden feelings, angry at his father for being the successful rival—and also angry at his mother for preferring his father. And it's the nature of a young child, if he feel jealous and vengeful towards his father, to assume that his father has just the same jealous and vengeful feelings towards him. Realising that his father is so much bigger and stronger, he dreads what might happen if his father ever let his anger out.

Studies of the unconscious show that a boy is apt to have particularly strong feelings of rivalry about his father's much more impressive genital equipment and to fear that his father's anger may be directed against his (the boy's) penis. This genital focus of his anxiety results partly from the boy's earlier worries about physical differences between boy and girl and about injury from masturbation. These are

19

the main factors that make the boy repress his romantic feelings for his mother.

The girl at this stage wonders if the romantic rivalry between her mother and herself is to blame for her own lack of a penis.

These fears eventually take the pleasure out of the small child's romantic daydreams and make them seem unpleasant instead. (Feelings about other matters can be reversed in the same way. Love of a certain food may be changed to disgust if a person becomes sick soon after eating it. Love of a place may be changed to aversion if a terrible accident occurs there.) The result is that by the time a boy is about seven or eight years old, he doesn't like to think romantically about his mother at all. Most of the time he doesn't even want her to kiss him. By nine he is apt to have an aversion to all girls. He calls them silly or disgusting. He groans when there are love scenes in movies or on television.

Because of these worries a child is less likely to get involved in sex play with other children between six and eleven years of age, or to play with his own genitals, especially if he has been brought up in a strict family.

A girl now gives up much of her romantic interest in her father and tries to suppress her interest in sexual and romantic matters generally. However, most girls don't develop nearly as much awe of their mothers as boys do of their fathers. Girls can go on being physically affectionate with their fathers. They don't usually feel that boys are disgusting at eight and ten, though they find them pests all right.

This story of rivalry and fear and aversion probably sounds strange and unlikely. It does to most people, unless they've worked in the field of psychoanalysis and have seen the evidence for themselves. You have to remember that the antagonisms and fears I've been describing are in the unconscious layers of the small child's mind. He still admires and loves his parent of the same sex in his everyday existence.

Interest in God, Science and the Three R's

What happens to these romantic attachments and drives when they are repressed after the age of six or seven? The great admiration the children used to feel for their parents now goes out to the faraway heroes of books and comics and TV programmes. Much of their respect and awe is now transferred to civil authorities such as policemen, the Queen, the Prime Minister, and also to clergymen and God.

Their interest in where babies come from, in the mysteries of their bodies and in the opposite sex is sublimated into a fascination with the impersonal mysteries of nature and science. (The sublimation of primitive drives means that they are transformed into interests which are much more acceptable to society.) And one reason children become so eager to learn reading and writing and arithmetic at this age is just that these subjects *are* impersonal and abstract; they help them to get their former preoccupation with parents and love and sex and babies out of their minds.

As children try to be more independent of their parents, they sense the need to become more conscientious, more law-abiding, all by themselves. They get interested in rights and wrongs and rules. The games they now play don't any longer have to do with imitating their mother's and father's daily activities, but rather are concerned with skills and rules, as in games like hopscotch. They now enjoy being systematic; this explains their fascination with collecting such things as stamps, cards and rocks. They form secret clubs so that they can practise being responsible citizens all by themselves, far from adult supervision.

You can see that this age period between six and eleven years is given over to learning how to control your instincts and how to conform to the society outside your family.

It is interesting that a child's body grows much more slowly during this stage (he will grow rapidly again at the beginning of adolescence), as if full growth and strong instincts are both being postponed for a number of years, until the individual has learned to control himself and to respect the complicated rules of human society. Other animals don't have any such separate stage of development, physically or psychologically; they keep increasing rapidly in size from birth right up to maturity.

Puberty and Adolescence

What eventually puts an end to the middle period of childhood is the abruptly increased activity of the sex glands (ovaries and testicles) in the puberty stage of development which introduces adolescence. The glands now make the body grow at a much faster rate. They enlarge the genital organs and start them functioning. They bring out the 'secondary sex characteristics'—pubic and axillary hair in both sexes, breasts in the girl, beard and voice changes in the boy. (These are discussed in Section V.)

The previous repression of sex and romance cannot disappear suddenly. Boys are torn between interest in girls and embarrassment when near them. Girls do not have as much inhibition to overcome, but even they are made very self-conscious; some become painfully shy; others find themselves showing off in a noisy way that they didn't intend.

Because the repression of interest in the opposite sex has been so strong, the intensified personal feelings caused by the glandular changes often go out at first to members of the same sex, especially to admired adults such as teachers.

A boy may also feel attraction towards an actress or entertainer whom he can love and dream about to his heart's content at long distance, without having to worry about whether he has the sophistication to carry off a real date. A girl may become infatuated with a remote male idol.

Or the teenager may fall secretly in love with an appealing adult of the opposite sex in his own community, perhaps because the adult seems more suave than those of his own age and easier to talk with.

Sooner in one case, much later in another, a young person of either sex finds himself falling in love with someone near his own age. It takes longer for him to find the courage to actually speak to his beloved and longer still to say anything important. (It wasn't until I was fifteen that I got up the courage to speak to the girl I had been watching in Sunday School since I was twelve. But all I could think of to say was 'Aren't you Marta Snead?')

People get over their shyness with experience. But for the shy ones it's so hard to get any experience.

Even when a boy's inhibitions have been overcome sufficiently to allow him to arrange a date with a girl, this does not mean, of course, that his whole sexual drive will now be directed towards the single aim of achieving a physical intimacy with her. There will be two other powerful expressions of it. First, the idealistic part of the drive which, back in early childhood, made him exaggerate and worship the spiritual qualities of his mother will now make him exaggerate and worship those qualities in his beloved. His

23

feelings for her will be tender and protective. He will want to win from the world the things she wants and to plan an idyllic life with her. This is sometimes called the chivalrous aspect of love.

Another part of his romantic drive, which was sublimated at about six years of age into impersonal aspirations to learn, discover, create beautiful things, perform great deeds, help humanity, will continue to be sublimated into these ideals— even for the rest of his life if he is a productive and creative person.

These ideals, which were relatively crude and simple back in the eight- or ten-year-old boy, are now refined by the youth's greater knowledge of the world and by his inner maturation. He can now not only dream about being a productive person; by the end of adolescence he may be able to be one. Many of the world's great literary works, musical compositions, paintings, scientific discoveries were achieved by young people just on the threshold between adolescence and adulthood.

Most animals will be attracted, during the mating season, to any member of the opposite sex who is near by. But the discriminating human adolescent or adult will automatically eliminate from romantic consideration most of the nearby members of the opposite sex because they are lacking in the bodily or personality traits that are important to him. That's the negative side. The positive side is the human condition called falling in love.

A boy will think of his beloved with emotions strong enough at times to make him feel dizzy. He daydreams for hours about imaginary conversations and experiences. His girl's beauty and charm seem fantastically great. He is thrown into depression if anything goes wrong between them, or even if he doesn't hear from her when he expects to. He feels sharp pangs of jealousy if she shows interest in

24

another boy. He is exultant when misunderstandings are cleared up or when he is about to see her again. A girl has the same feelings. A boy dreams of rescuing his girl from disasters or of going on quests or of achieving fame for her sake.

What is it that makes a young person able to feel romantically indifferent to a hundred members of the opposite sex of about his age, but fall head over heels in love with one? Psychoanalysts get evidence, from people's dreams and free associations, that what often plays a part in starting the infatuation is some characteristic of personality (perhaps combined with appearance) which can be traced back to the parent whom the individual loved so intensely in early childhood. That is what gives him the startling, breathtaking conviction, 'This is the one I've been searching for all my life.'

How Humans
Get their Attitudes towards Sex

My aim up to this point has been to explain how it is that a human being gets his basic feelings about the relationship between the sexes: it is not primarily from his glands but from the picture he forms of his parents' total relationship way back in the three-, four-, five-year-old period. It is not a realistic but an idealised image. He sees his father as an extraordinarily powerful, courageous, determined person who brings home the money he has wrested from others for the benefit of his wife and children. He sees that his father expresses his love for his wife and children in all the things he provides, in being dependable, in caring about their problems, in wanting to be with them. The father shows his very special love for his wife—as far as the young child can see—in having singled her out from all others, in being ready to fight her battles, in showing physical affection and tenderness towards her, in sympathising with her in her troubles, in being proud to be able to fix things and move things that are too much for her, in 'giving babies to her' (as small children are apt to express it), and helping her to take care of them.

The young child sees his mother as a beautiful, accomplished, and—particularly—a comforting person. She prepares food for her husband and children when they are hungry, finds warm clothes when they are cold, bandages them when they are hurt, reassures them when they are worried. She shows her romantic devotion to her husband by having chosen him above all others, by her pleasure at his attentions and physical affection, by her tenderness, her concern, her readiness to comfort him.

Every young child has this natural, inborn instinct to idealise his parents' love and devotion for each other—and also for him. If his parents during a quarrel threaten divorce, this will fill him with fear and he will implore them to stay together, for he senses that his total security comes from their devotion. He assumes of course that all sexual–romantic love belongs in marriage, because this is the only place he has seen it. The idea of a man and woman living together outside marriage or having an affair will not occur to him until his reading or his own feelings in adolescence bring up this possibility. When he gets into the six- to eleven-year-old stage, his sense that his possessive attachment to his mother has been forbidden by his father will further reinforce his belief that sexual–romantic love is only for parents. And since he will be proudly aiming towards this pattern for himself all through the formative years, it is no wonder that in adolescence and adulthood there still remains in his feelings a distinction between this 'normal' or honoured kind of married love and other sexual attractions.

I have been discussing how romantic ideals are passed from generation to generation in relatively happy families. But for contrast I can mention a couple of extreme, over-simplified examples of marital failure in which the child may end up with a distorted image of marriage. If a girl grows up with a mother who is a rather self-centred person who failed in her marriage, who dresses in exaggeratedly seductive clothes and can't help trying to attract the attention of all males (even though she may not have sexual affairs), the daughter is apt to get the basic sense that sexuality is mainly an exhibitionistic, seductive game. She may grow up to play a somewhat similar role; she may, on the other hand, acquire an exaggerated lasting revulsion against such attitudes.

If a boy has a charming father who irresponsibly deserts his family from time to time, he may be fascinated with his father's mysterious way of life and may eventually be drawn into copying him to a degree; or if his mother is a sensible person who depends on him for help of many kinds, he may later turn out to be an unusually responsible husband himself. The daughter of an unreliable gay dog may find him so appealing that when she grows up all the responsible young men will seem dull as dishwater and she'll respond only to a scoundrel; or she may be so dismayed by her mother's predicament that she'll never want to marry. The possible outcomes of any of these types of parental relationships are various and there is no predicting the exact effect on the children. I'm only making the point that the parents' marriage—whether it's ideal or impaired—has a strong impact on the children's expectations of marriage.

Why is Sex often Considered Sinful?

Now we can understand why sex is so commonly thought of as shameful, sinful or a subject for dirty stories and sniggering. Disapproving attitudes towards sex weren't invented by the older generation or by the Victorians. They can be traced back as far as recorded literature goes and occur in all parts of the world, though they've varied from place to place and from time to time. They result from the normal steps in psychological development which I've discussed earlier: the small child's assumption that sex properly belongs only to married couples, his anxiety about genital differences, any warnings he may have received about masturbation, his fear of the anger of the parent for whom he has feelings of rivalry.

Another root of disapproving attitudes is the closeness of his genitals to his annus and bowel movements, which he was taught, during toilet training, were dirty and naughty.

So the pleasurable excitement which used to be associated with his genitals and with daydreaming about his parent of the opposite sex before the age of five or six is changed to a sense of uneasiness about sexual love, particularly between son and mother, but also between daughter and father, and between brother and sister—the so-called 'incest taboo'.

Throughout the world—in civilised societies and in primitive societies—there are stern laws against a man's marrying his mother or his daughter or his sister. Usually the taboo applies to other close relatives, too. This feeling is so universal that we take it for granted. Yet other animals have no such aversion.

Also all over the world, men and women, however naked they are in other respects, cover up their genitals with some bit of clothing. And in the few places where they don't wear anything, men and women carefully turn their backs to each other when they pass on a path.

Many American children these days are raised in homes which are nudist colonies in spirit, because the parents have impatiently rejected modesty and the sexual guilt implied by modesty. Yet many of these children, when they become eight to twelve years old, will themselves demand privacy when undressing or using the bathroom.

Children of this same age raised by parents who deliberately try to avoid giving them any feeling of sin or dirtiness about sex nevertheless become uncomfortable when they watch romantic scenes in movies or witness earnest kissing between lovers.

Can't an educated person, when he finds out how primitive and irrational some part of his behaviour is—like shame about sex—overcome his irrationality by a deliberate effort of his mind? To a degree, yes. He can learn to talk about sex impersonally in a biology class. He can get used to going swimming nude in mixed company. But when he tries to override his deep scruples too far, he finds he can't go through with it or he feels uncomfortable afterwards. Man isn't that rational. His personality is put together on a moral–emotional framework. It certainly is true, though, that the scruples of one person or one group in society are a lot more easily overcome than those of another. I'm not trying to decide for anyone else what is right for him. I'm only explaining to those brought up with high standards the basis for their inner compunctions.

Why are so many adults—even idealistic ones—interested in sexual gossip, newspaper reports of love affairs, nude photographs, dirty stories? That interest is disillusioning to many teenagers, but it doesn't prove that the adults involved are perverted or hypocritical. When a child was three, four and five years old, his interest in *all* aspects of sex was free and lusty. On the one hand he greatly loved his parent romantically. But at the same time he was also interested in the physical, impersonal aspects of sex; he wanted to peep and could joke vulgarly about penises and breasts. Then came the inhibition of sexuality in the six-, seven-, eight-year-old period—an inhibition directed particularly against the love the child felt for his parent of the opposite sex. As a result it is the physical, impersonal and vulgar aspects of sex which come out of repression more easily. People get a sinful pleasure from letting anything out of repression, whether it's sex or hostility. They laugh at a vulgar sex story just as they laugh when someone slips on a banana peel. These crude aspects of man do not negate his aspirations towards idealism and kindness. They only show how complex his makeup is.

The Question of Sexual Freedom

The psychological theory of why there's a sense of guilt is less important for young people today than the ethical or personal question of how much sexual freedom is justified. Many of them, disgusted by the apparent hypocrisy of adults about sex, ask why sex should not be acknowledged as a wholesome activity in which any two consenting people should be able to indulge, as long as no harm is done to anyone. They believe that the discovery of 'the pill' removes the last block to such an attitude because it removes the fear of unwanted pregnancy and the shame the world imposes on an illegitimate child. This is an appealing picture—this picture of responsible as well as irresponsible people being able to enjoy sex as the spirit moves them, without having to worry about permanent obligation or hurtful consequences. Human beings have always had daydreams about this lighthearted kind of love. They have painted it into pictures of fauns chasing willing nymphs and have written it into countless stories of brief love affairs. Some people of course do carry these fantasies into action, at least for a while, particularly in their twenties, before they marry. It is at least temporarily satisfactory to some people, not to others. I'll point out certain of the factors involved, by comparing people who follow different courses.

The main trouble with fantasies of lighthearted love is that they take into account only the obvious desires and leave out the complicated and often painful truths. Most people who are emotionally grown up are not satisfied for long with casual affairs because—consciously or unconsciously—they are looking for someone to love deeply, to marry and to have children with; this has been their vision since early childhood. A great many of these individuals— especially those with high aspirations—have the ideal of saving sexual intimacy for the person they will eventually marry. (In saying intimacy I'm not specifying any particular degree.) Some keep this resolve, despite strong physical desire: others don't.

In these days of greater sexual freedom, there is a larger number than previously of young men and women, mostly in their twenties, who decide to live together before they feel ready to decide about marriage. Some of them later fall more deeply in love and eventually marry. Others separate because of an increasing sense of incompatibility; they find qualities that they don't like or too little of the qualities they thought they saw. A common cause of separation occurs when the woman has come to love deeply and is eager to marry the man, but the man has not become similarly involved and is frightened away by her wish for a permanent

31

relationship. This is an example, I think, of woman's romantic adaptability—her greater readiness to love the man who desires her, even when his desire is mainly physical. A man much less commonly falls in love with a woman just because she wants him.

When an affair breaks up, leaving one individual still in love, this may be extremely painful for him. And if he then tries to ward off later hurts by becoming shallow or cynical in his subsequent attachments, he may impair his capacity to make a sound marriage.

I think that the number of real sexual affairs nowadays has not increased nearly as much as the social acceptance of them; the people involved do not have to keep their relationship as well hidden today as they once did.

You may be interested to know that in Vance Packard's recent study* of the attitudes of today's American university students, a considerable majority of the men and an overwhelming majority of the girls expressed a conviction that intercourse was totally inadvisable before the age of eighteen except in marriage. And of these same students, nearly half the men and more than half of the girls had not yet had intercourse, though some of them were already engaged. You can compare these figures with those of the Kinsey Reports of twenty years earlier which showed that, of students, half the men and three-quarters of the women had not had intercourse. The shift to a much more permissive atmosphere about sex today, it seems, has resulted in only a moderate change in the actual sexual pattern for girl students and almost no change for boys.

* *The Sexual Wilderness*, Longmans Green, 1968.

The Relationship between Educational Level and Sexual Inhibition

The Kinsey Reports of a generation ago on sexual behaviour in America* showed that a majority of young people born in families with little formal education came to have intercourse relatively early in adolescence; the higher the educational level of the family, the older was the boy or girl, on the average, at the time of first intercourse. In many cases, especially at the higher educational levels, the first experience was during engagement or in marriage.

If the same study were made today, when sexual freedom is considered to be greater, the first experience would probably be shown to come somewhat earlier, on the average, especially for girls, in all educational groups. But it's safe to assume that those at the higher educational levels are still slower than those at lower levels to have intercourse.

In families of higher educational level the parents tend to be stricter about a variety of matters. They expect their children to go far in their education, and to do well at school in order to do so. They expect them—in their eventual careers —to reach a higher than average level of achievement. They tend to be very particular in their definition of good behaviour. More important, they try to instill high aspirations into their children's characters so that they will be *self-motivated* to be honourable and hard-working, even when they are thousands of miles from the parents. By contrast, a majority of parents with only an elementary education are primarily concerned that their children should simply not be bothersome while they are with them; they are much less inclined to think in terms of character-building

* *Sexual Behaviour in the Human Male*, W. B. Saunders, 1948; *Sexual Behaviour in the Human Female*, W. B. Saunders, 1953.

for the long pull or of working towards a life career.

A majority of parents with high aspirations for their children carefully foster the sublimation of the early childhood interest in romance, sex and having babies into scholastic and creative channels, whether or not they recognise that this is their aim. They (and the child's teachers) show their enthusiasm over his successes with his school work, they take him to museums, they are complimentary about his paintings, his stories, his block-building and his carpentry, they teach him respect for the authorities, they read to him about heroes.

I don't mean that these are better families—in my estimation or on any absolute scale; they are simply the families with higher standards and aspirations. It is of course relatively easy for a majority of the children of parents who have the educational and aspirational advantages to achieve equally high levels themselves. However, some of the world's great thinkers, leaders, creators and prophets have come from families with little education. (Biographies suggest that there was probably a mother, at least, in such families who had unusually high aspirations for her child.) And of course some of those born into families with all the advantages prove unable to profit from them.

There is an interesting postscript to this discussion which at first may seem an exception to the theme I'm discussing and yet really supports it. Kinsey looked into the small number of men who had lifted themselves by their bootstraps considerably beyond the level of their families—in education and career. He found that back when they were early teenagers, long before they got into a university or had any clear idea of the career they would eventually follow, they showed an inhibition of sexual behaviour which was like that of the people with whom they would later go to college and with whom they would be associated in their future jobs. So this is another indication that high aspiration and achievement is brought about—in part at least—through the sublimation of sexual interests in childhood.

Contrasts in Sexual Behaviour in Boys and Girls

The patterns of sexual behaviour of boys and girls, partly instinctual and partly learned, are quite different.

A boy takes a predominantly active role in finding the girl who appeals to him most and in persuading her to be his. But a large element in what makes a girl feel deeply enough in love to marry is *being* loved, *being* needed; so her part is, on the average, more passive. (Of course she plays a significant though subtle role in interesting the boy who appeals to her.) In physical sexual relations it is particularly obvious that the male role is more active, the female more passive.

For a boy or man the physical sexual drive is always on the surface or near to the surface, from childhood to old age. When an attractive girl passes near, the boy has an impulse to look, and he may imagine making some kind of advance. He is impressed by a girl's figure whether or not he knows anything about her character—or even if he knows that her personality in unattractive.

There is an egotism in almost all males which makes them, when they are talking with a girl, take it for granted that their attention to her is pleasing or even exciting, though they may actually be aged, unattractive or boring.

In any episode of lovemaking—cautious or bold, with new acquaintance or old partner—the strong instinct of boy or man is to keep progressing towards greater and greater physical intimacy, unless he is stopped decisively. In the case of a very timid boy, this progress may be so infinitesimal as not to be perceptible to an impatient girl, but the impulse is there, nevertheless.

In physical lovemaking, unless a man is totally self-centred and insensitive, a good part of his pleasure comes from arousing and giving pleasure to his partner. This does not come primarily from thoughtfulness but from instinct.

A boy or man is just as capable as a girl of falling deeply in love, of being faithful, of being considerate. But he can also, especially if he has no commitment to any girl, carry out a love affair based primarily on physical attraction in which his emotional involvement remains quite casual and which he can end with little regret on his own part, and even little concern for his partner. Boys and men, including those who are generally sincere people, are capable of vowing their deep love when making love or trying to make love to a girl who is still reluctant, even though they may feel little true love and are ready to make no permanent commitment; they are drawn into grossly exaggerating their love by their momentary enthusiasm for the girl's charms and by their own instinct to make progress in the seduction.

The attitude of a considerable majority of girls and women is quite different. Since they deeply desire to be loved and needed, the ones with warm, generous natures and good judgment will put up with quite a few handicaps in accepting husbands who convincingly need them—for instance, pompous husbands, unsociable husbands, awkward husbands, husbands who won't achieve great worldly success, husbands from scorned minority groups. This doesn't mean that women will accept any man who vows his love. They are quite realistic, more so than males, in recognising who will make a dependable, co-operative mate; they are not nearly as easily carried away as men (except perhaps in early adolescence) by a handsome face or fine figure.

On the other hand, the desire to be loved obviously traps many girls—especially the young and inexperienced ones—into believing that a boy loves them who may say he does (or says little) but who actually is looking for a predominantly physical affair. To put it another way, a girl is tempted to respond as a whole, loving person to a boy who, a more sceptical woman could see, is asking a lot but offering little.

A recent report shows that half of all college-educated women who had intercourse before marriage had it for the first time with men whom they loved to some degree and thought they might possibly marry. But only an eighth of college-educated men with premarital experience said they had had their first intercourse with girls they loved and expected to marry. This means, for one thing, that many women instinctively want to save the ultimate sexual intimacy for the man they expect to love for life, even in a period of great sexual freedom such as the present. The discrepancy between the figures for the women and those for the men also shows that some of these women expected to marry men who had no idea of marrying them. The figures re-emphasise the fact that boys and men much more often play the role of seducer and exploiter. A smaller proportion of girls and women are just as heartless, though.

Boys with consciences should realise that inexperienced girls can easily be taken in and hurt, and should curb their artfulness when it is not sincere.

In girls and women there is, on the average, considerably less sexual pressure. Most of them don't have an urgent impulse, when deprived of sexual outlet, to go on the prowl. There are exceptions, of course. A few girls and women are obsessed with sex, for complex psychological reasons. Girls at thirteen, fourteen or fifteen can be quite preoccupied and aggressive, romantically speaking, when the boys of their age are still backward.

Girls and women can be roused, step by step, to an ever-higher sexual excitement, and if experienced they may look forward to it. But they seem more able to wait at any level and to tolerate a cessation of lovemaking without having reached orgasm better than most men can.

By the time a boy or man has started making advances to his girl or to his wife, he is totally engrossed—unless there is an interruption. So he is surprised each time he discovers again that a wife or other long-time partner may be thinking of other topics, at least in the early phases of lovemaking.

One of the situations in which the two sexes commonly have trouble understanding each other arises when a girl or woman asks her long-time boy-friend or husband, 'Do you love me?' A girl may say this because she fears, consciously or unconsciously, that love is dying and she wants to be reassured, even insincerely. But this question is also fairly often raised in stable marriages. There is apt to be a touch of impatience in the man's voice when he says, 'Of course I love you,' because he thinks he proves his love by being a good husband or lover; but this isn't the tone or answer that the girl wants. Though women are more realistic than men in many spheres, they are nevertheless sentimentalists, ceremonialists when it comes to romance. It's to brides and their mothers in most cases that the marriage ceremony is intensely significant, not so much to the groom. It means a lot to women to have their husbands remember wedding anniversaries and birthdays.

Rivalry with Parents
and the Search for Identity

In adolescence comes the feeling that you want to be different from your parents, especially your parent of the same sex—for instance, in your taste in entertainment and art, in politics, in occupational choice—though you may still admire that parent for certain achievements. There are reasons for irritation too. You are aware that your parents seem to have things pretty much their own way—at least around the house; and your increasing size, strength and knowledge of what goes on in the outside world all give you a basis for feeling quite resentful at times at having to knuckle under to their authority, especially if they use it arbitrarily.

These strains are aspects of the rebelliousness of adolescence. A large part of this rebelliousness (psychoanalysts have discovered) is really a continuation of the rivalry that started between child and parent way back when the child was four, five and six years old—between boy and father, girl and mother. That rivalry is accentuated now by the fact that the child has, or soon will have, an adult-sized body, adult instincts, an adult anger.

If you are a boy, you realise that you will soon be a man, with a job, a wife and a home of your own, and it riles you that you are still considered a child in some respects by parents and society. If you are a girl, you know that it will soon be your turn to be the woman who attracts the men, accepts a husband and has the babies; this gives you the impulse to push your mother aside, though you may be much too polite ever to express this unless you are angry.

In simple societies this rivalry with the parent often comes right up on to the surface in the later adolescent years. It helps the young person to break free from his family for good. When I was a psychiatrist in the Navy in World War II, I had quite a few patients from the mountains of Kentucky and Tennessee, where people tend to be fiercely independent. The psychiatrist in evaluating each case has to get a life history which includes such things as how the young man first left home to go to work. Most of my mountaineer patients told similar stories about leaving home abruptly at fifteen or sixteen years old. A father would tell his son to do a certain chore. The boy wouldn't like his tone of voice or would consider the order unfair and he would baulk. The father would become angry and make a threatening gesture. The boy, without premeditation, would knock his father down. Then he'd realise that it was not suitable for a boy to stay at home after he had humiliated his father. So he'd turn on his heel, walk off to the nearest town and look for a job.

At the opposite end of the behaviour scale is the typical son of a professional man. Ever since he was a small child, he has accepted the obligation to do well in school as an essential part of the process of becoming a professional man himself—not only to meet his family's expectations, but also to be able to live up to and perhaps even rival his father's achievements. In this kind of family (and probably in yours), the father characteristically tries to be a reasonable, generous and encouraging leader to his son. If he feels impatience or scorn, he tries to suppress it. These attitudes in the father (when added to the boy's long training in conformity) make it difficult for the son to feel conscious anger towards him or to rebel, except for a little grumbling. To hit his father or even shout at him would be almost inconceivable. Psychiatrists have learned that the rebelliousness is there all right, but that it has to find indirect outlets and quiet forms. Many such boys remain respectful towards their fathers and shift all their irritation towards their mothers. They criticise their mothers' appearance and behaviour; they blow up when their mothers scold them or remind them of their unfinished jobs.

A fairly common sign of rivalry in families which value education highly is school failure—whether in school or university. The type of boy we are speaking of has the intelligence to succeed in school. He is the kind who wants to do well and go far in his education. He has done superior school work in the past. Yet suddenly he can't make himself study. Or he can't make himself write reports. Or his mind goes blank in examinations. Or his subjects don't have much meaning any more; they don't seem worth studying. In other cases, the student who has previously been co-operative becomes argumentative about everything in class or declines to follow instructions or is directly rude to his teachers or refuses to attend school at all. He is 'displacing' his rebelliousness from his father to his teachers. (I'm not talking here about the kid who doesn't believe in education at all or who has been a poor student or a truant all along.)

Sometimes school failure—especially in the university years—occurs when a boy first studies a subject that is related directly to his chosen career, particularly if he is thinking of following in his father's footsteps. If such a boy seeks psychoanalytic treatment, it sometimes becomes evident that he is failing in his studies because unconsciously he is afraid of competing with his father, just as the boy of five and six was afraid of competing with him. And the hidden, irrational fear may be either that he won't be able to do as well as his father and will then feel humiliated, or that he might do better than his father, who would then be furious and perhaps do him harm. (Remember that we're discussing *unconscious* fears whose roots date from the five-year-old period. Remember also that I'm not trying to diagnose everyone with a school problem, only to give examples of how subtle problems of some teenagers can be.)

School failure serves another unconscious purpose. It tortures the kind of parents who are particularly ambitious to have their child succeed. It's one of the most painful punishments a child can inflict on them. Yet he doesn't have to feel guilty because, whatever the reasons for his failure, they are all unconscious. Consciously he is trying as hard as he can.

Uneasiness about competing with the father may show up in another way. When a boy of sixteen or eighteen is asked what occupation he's heading for, he may answer that he doesn't know yet, that the only thing he's sure of is that his father's field (medicine, for example) doesn't appeal to him at all. Then at the age of twenty, the doctor's son may drop a remark at home about how much chemistry he's taking this year. 'Why so much chemistry?' asks his father. 'You have to, to get into medical school, of course,' the son answers. 'But I didn't know you were going into medicine!' exclaims the delighted father. 'Didn't I tell you?' asks the boy, in real perplexity. The boy has matured so much by the age of twenty that he is no longer unconsciously afraid of the competition implied in entering his father's field; yet the subject is still embarrassing enough so that he has forgotten to mention his change of plan.

Some forms of rebelliousness are productive, such as joining an unpopular reform movement. Others are only negative expressions of protest, as when young people wear soiled work clothes on formal occasions or go unwashed or keep their living quarters in an offensive turmoil; this is the messing mood that two-year-olds use when resentful.

Rebelliousness against parents is a natural, inevitable aspect of adolescence. It assists them in giving up the comforts and security of home, achieving real independence, working for progress.

The most basic problem for the young person, though he doesn't usually think of it in these terms, is to find his own identity, to find out what sort of person he really desires to be and to get started being such a person. This doesn't mean just the specific job he'll take or the hobbies he'll enjoy. It means the kind of personality he'll end up with, how he'll be thought of by his friends, family and himself. It's not so much a matter of coming to conscious decisions—it's gaining a sense of being an independent person, with a job to do.

There are three principal elements that go to make up the identity an individual finally achieves. First and foremost is the character he was developing all through childhood. A boy, beginning at about the age of three, has been striving to be a man just like his father, and the little girl to be like her mother. So they have had to cast themselves in the moulds of their parents—they are made of their parents.

But to become an effective adult an individual must break off most of his dependence on his parents, not just to become free enough to leave home, but to develop ideas and aims of his own so that he can help to solve the existing problems of the society in which he will live. His feelings of impatience and criticism towards his parents are what put him on the lookout for new ideas, new methods which may better solve the problems of the day—and incidentally also show up his parents' generation as pretty well stuck in the mud. How strong the rebelliousness in each individual is and what form it takes is a second element in determining his eventual identity.

The third element is the nature of the times and the needs of the times. These call on youth for different qualities in different historical periods. As Erik Erikson

43

explains in *Young Man Luther*,* the corruption of the church in Martin Luther's time, the real need for major reform, inspired in Luther a fearlessness, clarity, eloquence and perseverance of heroic proportions. In a less critical age Luther might have remained an undistinguished cleric.

Many of the advances of civilisation—technical inventions, scientific discoveries, new artistic directions and spiritual inspirations—have been conceived by young people just on the threshold of adulthood. Because they were impatient with the achievements of the past and because they had no need to defend the present, they were able to envision and bring on the future.

Today the world is faced with enormous problems. There are enough nuclear weapons to destroy the earth utterly—through brinkmanship or accident or insanity—yet they continue to be stockpiled and proliferated, with no hopeful plan for disarmament in sight. Wars, with weapons of new fiendishness, are causing death and desolation. Man has learned nothing yet about controlling his belligerence and suspicion.

There are now more hungry people in the world than there have ever been before. Yet there are technical means available—for the first time in history—for solving man's food and population problems. Tens of millions are sick unnecessarily. Hundreds of millions ask for goods and for productive jobs and for education. Only apathy, tradition, narrow self-interest stand in the way. The only hopeful sign is that a new spirit of impatience and idealism is appearing in youth. This may be just in time or it may be too late.

Just as important as acquiring a sense of who you are and who you want to be is to feel yourself integrated into the world you have chosen. You want to be accepted by some social group and some occupational group. You want con-

* Faber & Faber, 1959.

44

fidence that these people need you and would miss you if you disappeared. Those who have aspirations want to see a career ahead and to feel that they are on their way towards it.

There is nothing more frightening than losing your sense of identity and of belonging. Most individuals make the transition from childhood to adulthood, from the family to the world, gradually enough so that they never feel seriously detached, only uneasy at times. One strong comfort along the way may be a particularly close relationship with a friend who obviously enjoys you, is in tune with you, keeps seeking you. You have the assurance that if he sees this much in you, it must be there.

For modern young people who feel emotionally shaky, the psychiatrist's office or the guidance clinic may seem the sensible place to go. In communities in which there is no psychiatrist or clinic, a social worker may serve much the same purpose. Or a sympathetic teacher at school. A refuge for some is an unusually intense devotion to religion, including perhaps a close counselling relationship with one clergyman.

A majority of young people, by the time they are fifteen or sixteen years old, worry about the impression their parents will make on their friends and are slightly ashamed of them: when, for instance, their parents try to use teenage expressions and, more than likely, use them wrong; or when they tell anecdotes that they consider cute about the adolescent when he was a small child, or bring out old family photographs. Adolescents worry about the possibility that their parents will wear different clothes, or talk about different topics, or decorate the house differently from the way their friends' parents do.

There are several sides to this sensitivity. Teenagers are trying to graduate from being their parents' child and to become what they themselves want to be. They are still afraid that they will be judged in the world by what their parents are or do; the less conspicuous their parents are, the safer they will feel. More particularly, as they give up their old dependence on their parents, they have a compensatory need—a tremendous need—to be accepted more thoroughly by their own friends; they are apprehensive that their friends will assume that any peculiarity of attitude in the parent is shared by the child and might be a cause for rejection. Finally, though teenagers find their parents often diffi-cult or even infuriating, they do still love them and want them to be well thought of by their friends. (I remem-ber, when I was sixteen or seventeen, worrying most that my mother's hair just above the nape of her neck would come loose in the presence of my friends—as it often did—and straggle down over the collar of her dress. And when my parents came to visit me at boarding school, I dreaded that all the stray articles of clothing that hadn't got into the suitcases would be in a mess in the back seat of the car. These are examples of what small matters you can worry about at this age.)

For most young people this shame about the parents lasts a few years and then peters out. They acquire confidence in their own individuality and realise that they won't be judged in the world by what their parents are.

The Hippie mode of life is one of today's significant forms of identity crisis. The wearing of anti-stylish, inex-pensive clothes, the living in poor quarters, the revolt against working at commercial jobs, the communal sharing of meagre provisions, the group living, all are protests against the extreme materialism of the Western world today as well as ways in which youths can separate themselves from their parents—and irritate and alarm them. But in a constructive sense these young people are searching for a more spiritual life based on co-operation and love. Their philosophy is in some ways similar to that of the early Christians.

The use of drugs is in part an expression of the desire of young people to experience all sensations, including mystical ones. Espousal of free sexual love by some of them represents a contradictory mixture, I think. They want to experience sex, but many are not ready for a meaningful love between two people. They are protesting against the commercialisation of sex in advertising, theatre and literature, against the double standard and against the women who appear to grant themselves to men only in exchange for the material comforts of marriage rather than out of love.

I believe that nine-tenths of even those young people whose protest takes unusually negative forms today will eventually find productive roles in the effort to make a better world. In fact, particularly creative people have often been protesters rather than conformists in their youth.

The Meaning of Marriage

I explained what a solemn, important thing marriage seems to young children and why they assume that sexuality belongs within it. They look forward to having an ideal marriage like the over-idealised one they ascribe to their parents.

We know from everything we've learned in psychology and psychiatry that what young children dream about doing will continue to have a strong influence through the rest of their lives, no matter how much more sophisticated they may become later.

In adolescence, young people's picture of marriage may

47

no longer be consciously patterned after the image of their parents' union, since they are now often quite critical of the parents. (Unconsciously, however, its influence persists.) Now they are imagining what their own marriage will be, with a mate they already have in mind or an imagined one. Everything about the match is highly idealised, as it should be.

Americans seem generally realistic when compared with people of other nations; but there is one respect in which we talk and act as if we were quite naive: our almost universal credo that if a romantic infatuation hits two people hard, it's a sign that they were made for each other, are ready for marriage and will live happily ever after. This despite the fact that we have one of the highest divorce rates in the world! I don't mean that we are wrong to be optimistic or to believe in the power of romantic love. I only mean that we should balance and buttress this faith with a strong emphasis—on the part of parents, teachers and clergymen, and of story-writers for television, movies and magazines—on the realistic demands of marriage. For a majority of people, despite its pleasures and satisfactions, marriage is a difficult relationship, a difficult adjustment, which calls on all their maturity.

To the young unmarried person it may seem that the gratification of the sexuality of marriage would make up for, or cover over, a lot of personality conflicts. Not so. Sex is certainly a vital element in a great majority of marriages, which would be severely strained without it. (A small minority of marriages can be successful without sex.) But sex doesn't have the power to make people forget personality conflicts except for an hour at a time.

In many parts of the world, teenage boys and girls receive earnest instruction in how they are to conduct themselves as husbands, wives and citizens. They also learn of the serious obligations they will owe as a married couple to the family groups from which they come as well as to the tribe or nation. In other words, there is no pretence that marriage is just for romance or that the young couple exist for their own fulfilment. In some parts of the world a marriage is still arranged by the families on the assumption that the choice of a partner is too serious a matter to be left to the young.

There are many people, as you will find in any divorce court, who think of marriage as primarily a means of gaining something for themselves—such as material ease or sensual pleasure or escape from an unhappy home. These are people who have not grown up emotionally. Like children, they expect others to provide. They end up disgusted with their marriages because there are so many difficulties that come along with living with another person—selfishness, pettiness, rudeness, quarrels, slovenliness—unless there is a spirit of mutual devotion which helps both partners to recognise and overcome their faults.

In any *good* marriage each partner does *offer* aid and comfort and sensual pleasure to the other whenever he or she senses it is needed. But this is quite different from one demanding it of the other.

A way to define a superior marriage is as one in which husband and wife keep on trying to please each other with thoughtful co-operation, compliments, sympathy, remembrances, frequent gestures of physical affection—as they did during the engagement and pre-engagement phases. (It's one of the depressing aspects of human beings that often they devalue marriage as soon as they have achieved it.)

Another aspect of pleasing your partner is to be as attractively dressed (though it can be in work clothes) and well groomed for him or her as for any other person you particularly want to impress (for who else is half as important?), and to conceal yourself at times when you have to be unattractive (when greasing your face or using the toilet, for example). Some people will be surprised at these suggestions, believing that once you are married you are entitled to relax and be your thoroughly natural self. This attitude guarantees a humdrum marriage or worse.

In a superior marriage husband and wife not only love and respect each other for what they realistically are, but also each idealises the other, sees his aspirations, has confidence that the other will achieve his aspirations—and this faith of each helps the other to make progress.

When you are young, you take it for granted that parents are the people who are and should be always giving—care, comfort, clothes, pocket money, permission to use the car, presents, parties—though you wouldn't put it so crudely. It's characteristic of older people and mature people to be able to give a lot and ask for little. But even the most mature people must continue to receive love, understanding, approval and encouragement. This is what a happily married couple give to each other.

In an ideal marriage the partners carry out their roles with such charm, dash, warmth and originality that they inspire their friends and children to want to excel likewise. By cultivating their marriage they have made it into a work of art.

The greater part of the adjustments have to be made when the couple is first married. But even after ten and twenty years there are new challenges to be met: the births, illnesses, school problems and other crises in the lives of the children, the ups and downs of the husband's career and of the wife's outside activities and responsibilities, the illnesses, deaths and financial needs of other relatives. The sound family rises to each challenge, not without difficulty, and is further strengthened by it, the children included.

You may think that this last statement tries to stretch optimism too far. But I have seen families in which the children reached unusually high levels of understanding and responsibility partly because there was a brother or sister with a severe handicap whom they helped to care for. I have seen other families whose morale was permanently impaired because the parents were unable to rise to a similar crisis.

There will continue to be at least occasional quarrels in the best of marriages because husband and wife are still individuals, no matter how long they have lived together. And as long as they are intellectually interested in the world around them, they will be changed by it and then have to make adjustments to each other's changes. So it's not the frequency or the fierceness of the quarrels that is important, but the effort of the couple to avoid hurting each other deeply during fights and their readiness to make up afterwards.

Occasionally there is a person who hopes through marriage to solve a problem of his own—for instance, difficulty in settling down and tending to business, or a liability to fall in and out of love too frequently. Or he may hope to solve a problem of his intended partner—such as alcoholism. These are usually futile hopes. You rarely solve pre-existing problems by marriage. Usually you only add new problems and compound the old ones.

Teenage marriages can be stable or perishable. So can marriages entered into at any later age. The maturity of the people is more important than their years. But the statistical fact is that more teenage marriages collapse. This is a strong reason for girls in their teens to resist the panic that is common today if they are not married soon after leaving school or university. That's a silly, competitive style that has nothing to do with maturity or love. It's an invitation to trouble and disillusionment.

Patterns of Lovemaking

There is not much point in trying to describe lovemaking—whether it is hand-holding, embracing, fondling or intercourse. It is experienced as a matter of emotion and relationship more than action; so the words of even a poet or novelist won't come close.

Though we think of lovemaking as instinctive, as indeed it is primarily, the patterns of expression vary widely in different parts of the world. This shows that we learn many aspects of it while growing up—from books, movies and TV, from what we notice in parks and on beaches, from what we see our parents doing and not doing.

One of the most significant things brought out by the Kinsey Reports is the difference in the patterns of lovemaking at different educational or social levels in America.

The reports analysed all aspects of sexual behaviour in terms of educational levels. But of course Kinsey did not mean that sexual patterns are influenced directly by schooling. He used the extent of schooling as the simplest way to get at different patterns in various social and occupational groups. He distinguished seven educational levels, from those who had not even finished primary school, at one extreme, to those who had won advanced degrees in postgraduate work, at the other. And he found, on the average, progressive differences in sexual behaviour at each of the seven levels. Of course there were many individual exceptions to every conclusion he reached.

Earlier, I explained that, in families with higher education or higher aspirations (which tend to go together), sexuality is considerably more inhibited in childhood and adolescence than in families at simpler levels, and is more likely to be sublimated (side-tracked and transformed) into study-

52

ing, into dreams of romance and idealistic life plans, into scientific and artistic interests. The Kinsey Reports show that such inhibition of sexuality in childhood does not result in less pleasure when the young person comes eventually to full sexual expression, but actually results in a more elaborate pleasure. To be more specific, a majority of the couples who have had little education tend to progress rapidly, after only minimal embracing, to an intercourse which is quickly over, whereas a majority of those with considerably more than average schooling tend to draw out the preliminaries of lovemaking, in order deliberately to exploit the pleasures of various kinds of caresses for their own sake, and also to prolong intercourse.

In the more drawn-out lovemaking, lips, tongue, hands may make loving contact with lips, tongue, breasts or genitals—for several minutes or for many. Each couple after months and years of variation tends to settle on patterns which give the greatest mutual pleasure. A few couples even progress all the way to the climax of orgasm while engaged in the forms of lovemaking which most people consider only preliminary—because in this manner they reach ecstasy more surely or more pleasurably than by genital intercourse.

For most couples, however, the ultimate desire is for intercourse, in which the man inserts his erect penis into the woman's vagina. Her labia and vagina have been made more moist than usual by her excitement, so the penis can slip in more easily. The man has the instinct to thrust his hips rhythmically backwards and forwards to move the penis partly out and in again, to increase the sensation for both. Intercourse can last fifteen seconds; or a man can learn to hold back his orgasm so that intercourse lasts for fifteen minutes or more. As the couple come nearer to orgasm, both partners usually want the rhythmic motion to become more vigorous and the woman may participate in it too. At the moment of orgasm—and generous, experienced lovers try to make their climaxes come simultaneously—they are overwhelmed by five or ten seconds of intense, pulsating pleasure while the ejaculation occurs, and they cling tightly together. After orgasm there is usually a feeling of complete satisfaction and peace which often leads to sleep.

From a physical point of view, the orgasm of a woman is not as dramatic as a man's because there is no ejaculation, but emotionally the experience is at least as intense, perhaps more so. Many girls and women cry out during orgasm as if the emotion were too great to be contained.

Dozens of positions for intercourse are possible: face to face with the man lying more or less on top, supported on his elbows; or the man kneeling with the back of the woman's thighs against his abdomen; or both lying on their sides facing each other; or the woman lying on top or sitting astride. Or the woman can turn her back to the man, as she lies on her side or abdomen, or kneels up.

The frequency of intercourse among different married couples varies from once a night to once a month. An occasional man will sometimes want and be able to perform intercourse twice in a night. Most feel thoroughly satisfied by one episode. A majority of young married couples have intercourse one to five times a week. After the age of forty or fifty the frequency is apt to decrease, mainly because of the man's decreasing potency (ability to have erections). Man's ego being what it is, this decreasing ability will make one man try less often, make another try more often.

The first few attempts at intercourse tend to be disappointing for many people, especially girls, because there is so much awkwardness and anxiety to overcome.

Since men (like women) feel totally relaxed after orgasm in intercourse, they may assume that they are muscularly weak at such times too, and for a day or so afterwards. In fact many coaches ask their athletes to avoid intercourse before contests. There is no scientific basis for this assumption —it's just an idea which fits in with those underlying male fears of genital injury, loss of manhood, impotence.

Temperamental
Differences between the Sexes

This is a controversial subject. Some people earnestly believe that boys and girls are born with exactly the same temperaments and that any differences that show up later are due to the different ways in which boys and girls are treated. Ask other adults what they think.

Back in the nineteenth century it was assumed that boys and men had all the sexual drive, that girls and women had none. Now I think that we've swung a little too far in another direction. Many people assume that girls have instincts and interests which are exactly the same as those of boys, that the only inborn difference between the sexes is in the roles they play in producing babies.

I believe that there are basic differences in temperament at birth though I have no way to prove this to a sceptic. Then the parents and society treat boys and girls differently and this has profound effects.

Through the evolution of our species over millions of years, and most of it under hazardous living conditions, there have developed a division of labour between the two sexes and relative differences of physique and temperament to correspond to the two jobs. Of course there are also wide differences between individual males and females, some women having temperaments like the average man's and vice versa. I am describing what I think are average differences. Man is the fighter, the hunter, the performer of heavy work. He has to be able to pretend that he's not afraid or that an injury doesn't hurt. He is also the theoriser and inventor. He enjoys analysing a problem into its separate parts and then figuring out the solution. These characteristics make him, in most cases, a less sensitive, less personal, less emotional, more absent-minded type than the average woman. So he sometimes doesn't listen or understand when his wife is telling him something; or he may not even realise it when she is feeling upset. He has more ego than the average woman in the sense that he is afraid to admit that he has been wrong, afraid of losing face. Perhaps this is the main reason why, throughout the world, a man marries a woman who averages two or three years younger than himself—so that she will be more likely to acknowledge his wisdom and leadership. Partly because he cannot create a baby, as a woman can, he has a greater drive to create in substitute ways—as a builder of structures and machines, as artist, writer, composer. To be a good hunter or inventor he has also had to be the imaginative one, the bold one, the chance taker; otherwise mankind might never have utilised its potentialities for adaptation and survival, and civilisation would not have advanced. For the selection of a mate and in lovemaking the male by instinct takes the initiative and the more aggressive role. However, in most cases he is careful to estimate what his reception will be, to avoid the humiliation of a rebuff.

Boys and men have an instinctive need to prove that they are adequately virile—to prove it to others and to themselves. Under the surface there is some of this anxiety in all men. In the most secure males it is not noticeable on the surface. In the majority it is evident from time to time. In a few it is painfully obvious.

The male concern about virility takes many forms. In

the literal sense of sexual potency it is every man's wish and worry that his erections and his lovemaking be good enough to satisfy his partner. In a broader, more romantic sense it means being able to provide well for his woman (whether it's a mink coat or just a roof), to protect her, to impress her with his power or skill. In the widest sense it's being able to compete with other males—in jobs, income, size of car, athletic ability, courage, cockiness in standing up to another man in an argument or a bargaining session or a fight. The man's concern about adequate virility may seem pathetic or ludicrous, but it is one of the most powerful and useful motivating forces in our species. It keeps the productive machinery going, it brings about improvements in living and knowledge, it tones up the whole of civilisation. It is also one of the main causes of mankind's troubles. It makes men take crazy chances—in climbing mountains or driving cars or gambling, for instance. It makes some of them obnoxious in boasting, showing off or making unwelcome advances to women. It gets individuals into fist fights and lawsuits. It spurs national leaders to get involved in challenges which lead to war.

Though the male is designed by nature to be the more aggressive sex (with larger muscles and bones, for hunting and fighting), at the same time he has built-in psychological mechanisms by which his aggressiveness can be very effectively tamed, disciplined, sublimated, for purposes of civilisation. Take the extreme example of the gentle professor or scientist. It is likely that he grew up with thoughtful, conscientious parents who rarely if ever raised their voices against each other or him, and never their hands. When he began to play with other children, his mother was quick to stop him if he ever came to blows, and to urge him earnestly to share, to reason, to be fair and polite. He played mainly with children brought up in the same spirit. His parents, in their conversations, showed their admiration for individuals who excelled in scientific and cultural fields rather than in war or boxing. They showed great interest in their child's lessons, his progress at school and his projects. Partly as a result, he became a good student from the beginning in school. Throughout childhood his crude aggressiveness was consistently restrained; he learned to count on reasonableness to get what he felt entitled to. And the emotional energy which in the average male goes into vigorous occupational competitiveness, participation in sports and in following sports, sharp kidding, loud arguments and occasional fights, in him ends in all-absorbing intellectual pursuits.

In a comparable way the male's sexual drive can be effectively inhibited and sublimated to varying degrees during the childhood and adolescent years. It's a fair guess that, in the intellectual family I have described, the relationship between the parents contained a large spiritual component—tenderness, unselfish devotion, respect for each other's ideas and ideals. Probably the parents were restrained to some degree in their expression of physical affection in the presence of the child. The questions which the child himself raised about sexuality were answered in a dignified, intellectual manner, with emphasis on the biological facts and on the spiritual love between man and woman. Sexuality was not a matter for coarse jokes in this family. So the romantic and sexual drive was curbed and well sublimated into intellectual interests to a particularly high degree in the years from six to eleven. Even in adolescence, the restraints on sexuality are likely to make such a boy shy about dating for an unusually long period; that part of the sexual energy which was and is completely sublimated flows still into studying and scientific interests; that part of the sexuality which is only partly inhibited goes into daydreams about an inspiring girl in the future and the productive career he will carve out for her sake.

Woman since the beginning of the race has cared for the children, prepared the food, made the clothes, comforted and inspired her husband. So she has had to be aware of the feelings and personal needs of all the members of the family. The average woman is the sensitive, the intuitive one. She is the realist who copes with today's actual problems today. She is more often the conservative one— storing provisions, making plans for the future, ensuring the safety of the children—to balance her husband's risk-taking. She is usually more agreeable; as a student she doesn't need to argue with teachers as much as a male student does— either out loud or silently—and this is why she learns her lessons more easily and gets higher marks.

In expressing these opinions about the sexes, I don't mean for a minute that a woman can't be just as creative in science, literature, the arts, the professions or business as a man. She can be a theorist or an effective administrator. Some women can perform jobs that require aggression and daring. These outcomes depend on a combination of inborn temperament traits, on family influences and on aspirations kindled along the way to adulthood. I'm making the more limited point that a majority of girls start with less of certain temperamental inclinations compared to men, more of others. But if the girls are stimulated by an inspiring example or by strong competition, they can compensate for differences in original inclination. So can boys.

Rivalry between the Sexes
(Note : This is a controversial subject too.)

There is a normal tendency to rivalry between the sexes. A little girl at two and three comes to realise that a boy has a penis and she doesn't. The situation not only worries her for a while, but it makes her mad, because a very young child thinks it's better to have something than not to. It also makes her feel rivalry towards boys. Some girls and women keep this feeling of rivalry so intensely that it sours all their relationships with men—social, romantic and occupational. In others the rivalry is so slight as to be unnoticeable except at times of crisis. When it is strong, it tends to push women into activities and occupations in which they can compete more or less aggressively with men.

The rivalry of boys and men with women is based in part on the little boy's envy of a woman's capacity to grow babies. This is one of the factors that give more men than women, I think, a consistent urge to create things. Other men for this reason unconsciously attempt to outdo their wives in the care of the children or in winning the affection of the children.

I myself believe that the potential rivalry between the sexes is over-accentuated in America and some other Western nations by the way we raise children in the family and educate them in school.

In the less developed parts of the world boys are taught by their fathers, and perhaps by male teachers, how to prac-tise with pride and joy one of the few occupations that men carry out in that particular society. Girls are taught by their mothers to play proudly and enjoyably the part of a woman. (There are even fewer schools for girls in the under-developed countries than for boys.) Each sex's role is considered to be a vital and dignified one. The differences between them are accentuated.

In many homes there is relatively little difference in the way the parents treat their sons and daughters. They may dress them the same, much of the time, in blue jeans and sweat shirts, and expect them to play the same games together. They may assign them the same household chores. In school and university they study the same things, of course.

I'm not arguing that parents, teachers and children don't have the right to do things this way. But I think that treating the two sexes alike pits them against each other to some degree and increases the rivalry due to other causes. Women in America and parts of Western Europe during the past fifty years have increasingly been wearing clothes and doing their hair like men. Some of them now drink, shout, back-slap, use obscenities and tell dirty stories like men. In these respects I think they have been motivated more by rivalry than by natural inclination. To put it another way, what's so great about the way men do these things? Women have come into almost all the occupations once reserved for men and in the United Kingdom, Australia and New Zealand the principle of equal pay is accepted, but, as elsewhere, women are still unjustly denied equal access to all jobs, and equal consideration for promotion.

Women have the right to act any way they want to and to take any jobs they have the aptitude and training for. But the thing that I'm concerned about is that quite a few women nowadays, especially some of those who have gone to university, find the life of taking care of their babies and children all day boring and frustrating. I think that the reason is not that child-rearing is dull in itself. In fact men become pediatricians (children's doctors), child psychiatrists, child psychologists or schoolteachers mainly because they find it fascinating work to help children grow and develop; in a sense they want to do women's traditional work. I think that the main reason so many mothers are bored is that their upbringing and their education have made them somehow expect to get their satisfaction and their pride as adults from the same occupations outside the home as men.

One big trouble is that schools and universities don't teach about the tremendous contribution that women make to any society in raising the children and inspiring them to do great things. Schools and universities hold up for admiration the statesmen, generals, inventors, scientists, writers, composers and industrialists. So these are the careers that bright girls as well as bright boys dream of. When young women find themselves instead taking care of their children all day, some of them feel they aren't using their education, aren't being fulfilled. Some of them are resentful of the 'interesting lives' they believe their husbands have at work. I myself would say it is much more creative to rear and shape the personality of a fine live child than it is to work in an office or even to carve a statue.

Another reason why some mothers don't find mother's work rewarding is that many university-educated people come to assume that no job is dignified unless you had to take an M.A. or a Ph.D. degree to perform it. This is modern snobbery—not social snobbery but academic snobbery.

My prime concern is that, back at the childhood stage, parents and schools should not encourage girls to be competitive with males if that is going to make them dissatisfied with raising children, their most creative job in adulthood, whether or not they go to work too.

I believe that boys too should be brought up and educated to realise that rearing fine children of their own is *their* most important and satisfying job. It's crazy for fathers to get so wrapped up in their careers and committees that they have no time for their children.

There are several reasons why men may become unusually passive or domesticated. When a significant proportion of the women in a society become more competitive and aggressive, over several generations, they can push a proportion of the males into a more submissive role. It's hard to do that to an already grown man. But a bossy mother can train a lot of the spunk and spontaneity and manliness out of her son, beginning in infancy—forbidding him to play rough games or to play at all with rough boys, for instance, or stopping him every time he thinks up a project by himself. She can even make him slightly ashamed of being a male. Then, since a youth's marriage choice is apt to be influenced by the kind of relationship he had with his mother in early childhood, he may be more likely, when he grows up, to fall in love with a girl who has a lot of bossiness in her. (There will be plenty of bossy girls in such a society because girls tend to follow the pattern their mothers set for them.)

Another way in which some men have lost considerable sense of pride and masterfulness is by no longer being the only breadwinner in many families. In the olden days when only the man had an outside job and only he brought home the money, he and his wife thought of his function as unique and crucial—just as his wife's was crucial in the home. (Both of them had to work like dogs from sun-up to sundown in those days to get their jobs done.) Women in earlier centuries didn't even go to school. They weren't taught any athletic skills. Some women made their way in the world by exaggerating their helplessness. They let men feel all-wise, all-powerful, all-skilful. Nowadays, of course, women know as much as men, do well in sports that don't depend on bulk and brute force, equal men in many occupations and excel in some, even perform handyman jobs around the house. So men—whose egos depend on skill and prestige more than women's do—have been effectively deprived of their earlier sense of being uniquely important. I think that this has accentuated the envy of women they acquire at three or four years of age. As a result they have sometimes tried *unconsciously* to compensate by invading the wife's domestic area, doing a lot more housework and child care than men ever did before, even trying to outdo their wives in being fancier cooks, in being greater experts in child psychology, in being more popular with the children.

I don't want to give the impression that any time a man cooks or gives the baby a bottle he is competing with his wife. In fact a man can do one hundred per cent of the domestic work, when there is a good reason, without any implication of competition. The motive, not the act, is the significant issue.

As a result of the increased competitiveness of the female and of greater sexual freedom in general, many girls are becoming more aggressive in their relationships with boys. When you see them on dates, in public and semi-public places, it often looks as though it were the girls who were making the advances. Attractive school and university boys tell of being pestered by frequent romantic telephone calls from girls they know only slightly. On several occasions when, in speaking at universities, I've mentioned my impression that many girls are becoming increasingly aggressive romantically, the men in the audience have expressed vigorous, disapproving agreement. Things like this didn't occur twenty-five years ago. You may answer with the age-old saying 'Other times, other customs' which means, correctly, that the world keeps changing, and who is to say that what used to be was better? I agree it would be possible for the human race to continue to exist with women taking most of the occupational, romantic and sexual initiative. I'm only suggesting that in the long run this would make both sexes less and less happy. When women become regularly dominant, males lose much of their eagerness for the chase and a lot of their sense of masculine dignity.

Occupations for Women and Men

The human being differs from all other species in his extraordinary adaptability to various styles of existence. There is no one occupation that can be called normal for women aside from gestating (growing) babies in the uterus. Women have been farmers, novelists, dancers. As rich men's wives they have sometimes left all useful feminine functions to servants. In ancient Crete they fought bulls, with breasts bare.

Man has taken to an equally wide range of work. He has been warrior, merchant, poet, physicist, religious mystic.

Since World War I, when they were needed in defence industries, women have increasingly been going to work outside the home. That period helped to break down the feeling of husbands that it was a reflection on their capability as wage earners if their wives worked. World War II gave another big boost to the trend. More and more jobs not requiring brute strength have been developed by our complex society. The hours of the workday have been progressively decreased. Employers have provided part time jobs so that mothers could get the breakfast and supper at home and still put in nearly a full workday outside, or even work only a few half days a week.

Today's mother is much more likely to be still young,

energetic and interested in a job when her children are all well started in school than her grandmother was. Back at the turn of the century the average age for marriage for women was twenty-six. They continued to have children from then until they entered the menopause at about forty-five. So they were often in their fifties before their youngest child reached the third or fourth year at school—not an age when many women are eager to take on an outside job, after staying at home for thirty years.

Nowadays women marry so much younger and plan their children's births so efficiently that half of them have had their *last* child by the time they are twenty-six. This means that if they want to take a job when the youngest is in the third or fourth year at school, they'll only be in their mid-thirties. No wonder so many are looking outside the home for a place to be useful and for fulfilment.

This trend will probably continue. I think that's fine as long as children can count on a loving mother's being at home most of the time until they are seven or eight years old.

What about mothers who are interested in having full time jobs even when their children are babies? Some people advocate that nurseries be provided at public expense where any woman could leave her baby during the day from birth onwards and that public nursery schools be available for children three years and older. Such systems have been used with reasonably good success in Israel and the Soviet Union. We have had a limited number of nursery schools in America for years—private and public—and will undoubtedly have more. In Britain the number of nursery schools provided by local education authorities has increased greatly in recent years as public opinion has prompted the Government to find more funds for this purpose. This has been matched by a rapid growth in the number of play groups, provided and staffed by volunteers. The *nurseries* we have had for a hundred years in America for children between birth and three years of age have been mostly of low quality, run by untrained people, and have often turned out children permanently impaired by emotional neglect. In Britain the public concern about the low quality of some of the care given to children of working mothers by 'baby-minders' has led to regulations providing for registration and inspection of premises used for such purposes. Many employers now provide nurseries for the children of mothers who work for them.

In the Soviet Union and Israel women of warm character and suitable training are proud to care for other people's children, as a contribution to the nation's welfare. In America and increasingly in much of Western Europe women are glad to work as *trained professionals*—in psychology or teaching, for instance—but it is very difficult to recruit them for simple, loving, maternal, non-professional care of infants and children, such as house-mothers give in institutions for neglected or physically handicapped children. This is partly because the pay of a housemother is less than that of a psychologist. But I believe that low pay is less important than low prestige, based on the assumption that because no special education is required, no significant contribution will be made. A woman medical student in a class of mine said, during a discussion of this topic, that she thought full-time motherhood would be a boring and frustrating job, but not child psychiatry. When I asked why, she declared impatiently, 'The psychiatrist is trying to *accomplish* something!' I myself would estimate that a good mother or father can accomplish more for the good of society than a psychiatrist.

Another problem in setting up nurseries for the care of very young children of working mothers is that there must be only three or four babies per caretaker, in order to give them the feeling of being loved as individuals. That means that the government would have to hire and train one woman to take second-rate care of the young children of perhaps only two mothers at a time—an expensive, inefficient system.

Most significant to me is the fact that in the crucially formative period of early childhood, it is the character and attitude of the person who spends most of the time with the child which largely determine the basic and special qualities of the child's personality—whether he will turn out optimistic or pessimistic, trusting or suspicious, loving or withdrawn, creative or conventional.

Psychoanalytic studies of that small minority of individuals who have been extraordinarily creative in the arts and sciences show that they had been inspired by a strong relationship with a mother who had particularly high aspirations for her children. For myself I would say, 'What is the gratification of being a parent if I am not to be one of the most influential people in shaping my child's character?'

It is known to be definitely harmful to a baby or small child if the caretaker on whom he has developed a real emotional dependence leaves him—and this is intensified every time such a loss is repeated. This introduces a special hazard in substitute care, especially in America where people move so often.

I'm all for good nursery schools for children of three and four, whether or not the mother wants to work. But to be good, schools must be expensive—to the family or to the state. Someone must be available to care for the child at home when he is sick—which is often, at this age. And most teachers and psychiatrists consider it desirable, if at all possible, that the mother resume care of the child by midafternoon.

Some young couples attempt to find jobs at staggered hours so that father and mother between them can take full care of their babies and small children. This plan will take care of their child's emotional needs but may prove difficult for the parents to arrange and maintain. A few couples are discussing or experimenting with raising their children in a commune of several families, so that one or two mothers who want to work can regularly leave their children with a mother who doesn't. Whether such an arrangement would be sound for the children would depend very much on the emotional stability of the substitute and the stability of the group. The primary attachment of a child under three should not be interrupted.

My own conclusion from pediatric experience has been that it is difficult for a mother to work *full time* and still find a way to do justice to children under the age of seven or eight. The commonest compromise, for those who are eager to work, is to work part time—two or three half days a week, for instance—while a husband, grandmother or reliable, loving sitter minds the baby. By the time the young child can be in a nursery school, the mother may be able to go to her job half or three-quarter time.

What I'm primarily concerned with is the spirit in which girls and boys are brought up in childhood and youth. I believe that if a girl is raised at home and taught in school to have pride in the creativity of motherhood, joy in being a woman, a sense of fulfilment through her ability to understand and help people, she will be happier as a wife and mother. And then if she has an outside career in addition, whatever it is, she will bring her womanliness to it. As a physician, architect, teacher or lawyer, she will be able to help humanise these professions—to counteract the common masculine inclination to focus on theory and form and detail. In other words, she won't feel that the main satisfaction of any career is to compete with the men at their own game.

Boys should be raised with as much anticipation of fatherhood as of an outside job, and with a conviction that they can be manly, courageous, inventive, and still show tenderness and understanding.

I myself would like all school and university students—boys as well as girls—to be reminded often that in all probability their most creative work as well as the job that will give them the greatest satisfaction in the end is bringing up fine children, loving them, being proud of how they turn out. Young people would believe this more if it came from teachers than if it came only from parents. There should be courses in family life and child development in all schools and universities. There should be nursery schools in all secondary schools and universities, where young people can get practice and achieve wisdom in taking care of children.

[II]

Boy–Girl Relations
in the Teens

The Contrast between
Romantic Love and Physical Sex

An uncomfortable problem for you as an idealistic young person, especially in the early teens, is the sharp contrast between the physical side of sex and the romantic, tender, spiritual side. By the time you are in your late teens or early twenties, these two aspects will tend to fuse together (sooner in one individual, later in another), giving strength and meaning to each other. But at first they are so opposite that they seem to battle against each other.

The physical aspects of sex are crude and insistent, especially in the teen years. They will not leave you alone for long. They suggest to your imagination physical intimacies which are exciting or shocking. They prod you constantly to go where there might be members of the opposite sex—to look and to be seen. They make you try to attract attention before you know what you are doing. They push you into situations—whether you're pretending to be helpful or just fooling around—in which there is an excuse to touch a person of the opposite sex who appeals to you.

If you are a boy and are alone with an attractive girl, there may be an insistent preoccupation with the thought of making advances of some kind. (When I say making advances, this may mean as little as trying to hold hands.) In your first year or so of dating there may be very limited enjoyment of the relationship because you are so preoccupied with the question of whether the girl considers you timid for being so slow or whether she thinks you are obnoxious for being so fresh. And are you only going to try to hold her hand or are you going to put your arm around her, or to kiss her, or to be even more aggressively bold? If you are a girl there is the corresponding preoccupation about whether to invite an advance—by a subtle remark, by a look, by letting your hand touch the boy's arm or your knee touch his. All of this may have little to do with affection. It's partly your glands, applying their pressure. It's also the impulse to master a new ability. Human beings—from birth onwards—feel the challenge to master any new skill which confronts them, whether it's the physical skill of walking, the mental skill of reading, or the social and emotional skill of dating.

In the first few years of dating, the compulsion to make advances is a rather cold-blooded and promiscuous thing in most cases. By cold-blooded I mean that often there's little affection or respect for the other person. By promiscuous I mean that the teenager may have the impulse to make at least slight advances to almost everyone of the opposite sex who appeals to him at all, if the opportunity arises and if he has the courage to try. He may be quite in love with one person and yet be making advances to others.

Falling seriously in love is a different process. It sometimes comes on gradually, with the dawning realisation that a person you've known for a long time now means something very special. More often it starts with a pang of excitement on first meeting, followed by an increasing sense of infatuation. By infatuation I mean you feel swept along, dizzily, happily, in an all-absorbing involvement, much too turbulent to analyse, to control or to resist. It can peter out or it can continue to grow. It peters out when further acquaintance reveals to the couple that there is no real basis for attraction, no common interest. It strengthens into true love when time shows that the two have more and more to share, that they want to give to each other more than to take, that

73

each person supports and complements the other in a way which enhances his joy in life and his effectiveness.

When two people are gradually falling more deeply in love, their physical desire for each other keeps increasing too. In the case of most couples, the girl's desire is less insistent. Also, a girl who has depth to her character would like to be sure at each step that her love and her boy-friend's love seem to be permanent before she yields further intimacy of body and spirit. So she characteristically is the one to impose restraint. And the boy, because his love is tender and respectful, accepts the limits she imposes. So physical intimacy follows and is controlled by love.

The sequence is different when physical attraction and experimentation take the lead from the start. Two young people are attracted to each other; what kind of attraction is not yet clear. It soon turns out that there is not a tender, generous responsiveness between them, a hope that this might be the ultimate love. But there may still be a strong attraction, based on some combination of appearance, seductiveness of personality, glandular pressure and the impulse to experiment with sex and to master the art of it. In affairs such as these, the excitement of each stage of intimacy creates an increased desire for a further stage, with no other feelings strong enough to impose restraint. This sequence may lead to intercourse after a few months, sooner if either of them has had previous experience, or to other intimacies that young people sometimes refer to as 'everything but'.

What happens in the end to these predominantly physical affairs? They may proceed excitingly for a while, particularly among couples who do not have high aspirations for themselves; but such relationships rarely last for very long, because they fail to satisfy the human longing for a truly loving union. And young people who are sensitive and who have ideals tend to become at least mildly disgusted with themselves and with their partners when they are using each other's bodies mainly for physical gratification.

When I contrast the relationship in which increasing love takes the lead and keeps physical intimacy subordinated to it, and the relationship in which physical desire and experimentation are the chief motives, I'm oversimplifying, of course, by taking examples from both ends of the scale. There are thousands of kinds and combinations of human relationships. I don't mean that the idealistic young person (the person I also describe as having aspirations or high standards) always keeps away from the predominantly physical affair. The drive that comes from the glands and from the compulsion to experiment and master is just as intense in the idealist as in anyone else. But if he does have dates that are predominantly for physical gratification and experience, he will probably come to them when he is older than average and he will be more cautious during them.

My purpose in contrasting two types of involvement is not to moralise or to advise. Each individual has to work out his own philosophy and behaviour depending on his ideals and what he learns from experience. I want to explain certain aspects of human nature and how they vary in individuals brought up in different ways, so that you can better understand your own situation and learn how to be most comfortable during this turbulent period.

I'm focusing more on the situation of the idealist because he is the one who has more inner conflicts and is more anxious for explanations.

Early Dating and Going Steady

I don't think that the recent trend to earliness in dating and in going steady and in sexual intimacy means a readiness to share love, in a great majority of cases. In past generations in America, as well as in other Western societies like ours which are committed to advanced education, a great majority of young teenagers with aspirations were satisfied for a couple of years to be in love from a distance most of the time, with only occasional encounters; they did not become heavily involved until their late teens. The new trend has been primarily a style, I think. I'm raising doubts about it because I think that these recent customs give young people who are not yet ready to make choices that last or to love deeply the impression that sexual–romantic love is essentially physical in nature. And when thirteen-, fourteen- or fifteen-year-olds go on regular dates in which they can have privacy, the temptation to fill the gaps in the conversation with exploratory, physical sexuality will be great and will increase from date to date.

When going steady has become the custom among a majority of young people in a community, the custom in itself puts pressure on the rest to do likewise, in order to conform. Having a steady boy-friend to take her to all parties provides a girl with great security; it makes her one of the successful girls and she is never embarrassed by being stranded in public. These social advantages have often caused girls, they tell their teachers and doctors, to give in to the demands of boys for more physical intimacy than the girls would otherwise have granted.

When I say that few young teenagers are yet ready for deep relationships, I don't mean that they don't have strong emotions. The feeling of love for someone may be over-

76

powering, just as intense as anything felt at an older age. But usually the emotion proves not to be based on mutual knowledge and affection but on the appealing appearance of the other person and fantasies about what he is really like. The one who is infatuated often has no idea whether the other will reciprocate, whether the two have common interests, whether they can mean anything to each other and give anything to each other. This is why so many young loves blaze brightly and then burn out in a few weeks or months. The absence of a solid foundation for such a relationship has given rise to the expression 'They were in love with love.'

Sometimes a physical intimacy has begun to develop during the initial infatuation. Then as the romantic aspect of the infatuation begins to subside because of the lack of substance behind it, the young couple may substitute an increasing physical intimacy, to conceal from themselves for a while the failure of love to develop.

Dehumanisation of Love in America

An American medical student I knew who had spent a year in a European university after graduating from a college in the United States told me that he had been immediately struck by the different attitude of late adolescents and young adults he knew in the European country towards dating and romance: when a young man there becomes seriously interested in a girl, he acts visibly excited, elated, 'in love'. Lovers when separated are obviously thinking of each other, anticipating reunion. While on their dates, they look joyful and worshipful. They may bring flowers or simple presents for each other and write poetry if they are able.

This full acceptance and expression of tender and romantic love made the American realise for the first time how much this aspect is omitted in his country, how much of dating is given over to physical sexuality—and also to endless talk about how far to go, as if the couple were impersonally discussing hygiene or psychology in a classroom.

This is of course an unfair exaggeration, for there are many young Americans who are romantic about their beloved, and lovingly respectful of each other's bodies. But the medical student's observation supports my view that the encouragement of early dating before young people are mature enough to know what their ideals in life are, before they are able to think in terms of each other's emotional needs rather than their own desires, before they have a tender love to offer, has a tendency to dehumanise love and is a poor preparation for marriage.

Illegitimate Pregnancy

While we are talking about the experimental, physical kind of sexual affair which fairly often goes on to intercourse nowadays, without any real love, I want to speak of illegitimate pregnancy. Many people assume, now that there are 'the pill' and other efficient forms of contraception, that unwanted pregnancies don't occur. This is not so. In fact illegitimate pregnancies have tripled in the United States in the past twenty years. You wonder why it happens. In one type of case the boy and girl say it was because 'one thing led to another', without the young couple's ever having planned it that way or taken any precautions. They may firmly decide that it was all a mistake, that they won't let themselves do it again and so won't have the need for any contraceptive. Yet they may succumb repeatedly. Such people are quite immature. Those with a sense of responsibility manage to control their feelings. Or if they make the very serious decision to carry on an affair, they carefully take the precautions.

In another type of situation, a much more common one, a girl involves herself in an affair, not carried away by love or passion but almost coldly, with a man who means little to her, and still takes no contraceptive precautions. When a psychiatrist or social worker is later trying to help her find out the psychological meaning of her pregnancy, so that she won't repeat the tragedy, it often turns out that she has been very hostile to her father and mother—feeling that they have been unfair and unloving to her—and that, in the unconscious layers of her mind, she had permitted the pregnancy to occur as a way of embarrassing and shaming them in the community. Of course in hurting them she hurts herself much more. This is why the psychiatrist calls her act a neurotic one. You wouldn't believe that people who are otherwise intelligent and sensible could punish themselves so harshly, unless you had worked professionally with such problems.

Some of the girls who let themselves be easily involved in physical affairs without love or meaning and who then carelessly become pregnant are individuals who simply don't think much of themselves and don't expect others to think much of them either. When a man wants to make love to them, they are pleased to think that perhaps they are more attractive than they had realised. To put it another way, the girl with self-respect doesn't throw herself away and threaten her whole future in a shallow affair.

Some young people think that an illegitimate pregnancy doesn't have to be a serious problem in these tolerant days. I believe that they are mistaken. The talk is a lot more permissive today. But the girl who has to go through with a pregnancy will find that the secrecy still has to be as strict as in former times. The neighbours and relatives will be almost as suspicious and almost as disapproving. The girl and boy themselves will lose a lot of the respect of their friends. More important, they will lose a lot of their self-respect. Some young people think that by refusing to take the pregnancy too seriously themselves and by laughing off the neighbours and relatives as old fogies, they themselves will be able to brush off the disapproval. But it's impossible for anyone, unless he has an elephant's hide, to ignore that much criticism. Either the boy and girl will feel depressed and ashamed for a long period, or they will have to become cynical as a defence against the disapproval. Neither attitude is comfortable to live with. The cynicism, if it goes deep, can interfere very seriously with a person's career and his happiness in life.

If there is true love, a hurried marriage will solve a majority of the problems. But it is too bad to begin a marriage and a baby's life amidst the raised eyebrows and sniggers of the neighbours.

If there is little love between the boy and girl, deciding the marriage is the only solution will tend to foster cynicism in the couple—about themselves and about matrimony in general.

Life will be harder on the baby than it should be, whether he merely has a birthday embarrassingly close to his parents' wedding, or has to make his way through childhood without a father or even a father's name, or be adopted.

The Question of Petting

Roughly speaking, there are two kinds of dates, at least from a boy's point of view. In one he feels drawn to a girl primarily by her physical attractiveness (which includes a certain seductiveness of personality) and will go as far as he has the boldness to try or as the girl will permit. In the other he is attracted by a girl's whole personality, including her physical appeal, and wants to know her better; somewhere in the front or back of his mind is the thought that this might possibly turn out to be *the* exciting relationship of his life.

In a girl's feelings also there are the two kinds of dates. But there is lots of evidence that a girl doesn't distinguish so sharply and calculatingly as a boy; she tends to hope that any kind of dating relationship will turn into true love.

In a logical sense there should be no need, during the first few dates between a boy and girl who feel drawn together primarily by a liking for each other, for the boy to attempt any physical advances; their main pleasure should be in getting to know each other better, talking about tastes and opinions. The fact is, though, that most boys and men not only have the desire, but on a date with a new girl feel an obligation to try, so that if she is expecting this she won't find them too timid. This will be particularly true of a teen-ager who has not gained much experience or assurance yet in getting along with girls. In his first few dates with a girl, before it is really clear what the relationship is to be, he will surely feel a combination of urges, even if he doesn't succeed in making the slightest move. (The word 'advances' as I use it may mean anything from hand-holding to kissing and embracing to fondling.) There is the simple, instinctual, physical desire to make some sort of contact and, if that is

81

achieved, to try constantly to make further progress in physical intimacy. There is a gnawing curiosity in the inexperienced person to find out what sexuality consists of in all its forms. The most compelling drive of all, in the adolescent boy, is to prove his virility and masterfulness—to himself and to the girl. I don't mean that he has to go far to prove himself at first. Just to have arranged the date or to have succeeded in holding hands may seem great triumphs. But how to prove himself to the girl is a more baffling, haunting question.

Though a boy usually takes the initiative—or assumes that he should—actually it is the girl who, sooner or later, has to indicate to him what she considers appropriate or satisfactory. For example, by showing in a clear but friendly way, in response to the boy's cautious advances, that she is happy to let him put his arm around her waist but that she does not want to let him kiss her (at this stage, anyway), she not only keeps the intimacy at the level which seems right to her, but also reassures the boy that his virility has been entirely adequate to the occasion—that he would only prove himself an oaf by trying to go further. With this reassurance he can then do his part in carrying on a conversation about other topics and in making progress in companionship.

I've made it sound here as if only the boy was in a turmoil and as if the girl was as cool as a cucumber. This isn't true, of course. She has her own desires, her own curiosity about sex and love, her own deep need to be proved attractive and lovable, all of which are particularly insistent in the early teens, before she has learned from experience that she has what it takes. So it is difficult for her to say no in the 'clear but friendly way' I mentioned. If she is not clear, if she is hesitant, the boy will realise this and will feel that he is expected to be more bold and persistent. I said 'friendly' because it isn't necessary in most cases for the girl to act

shocked or indignant or angry. Most boys, in dating, are
sensitively attuned to the girl's attitude and will respond
promptly when she makes her feelings clear. If you reproach a boy too sternly, you may make him feel more
guilty than he justly needs to be. However, a girl may have
to be severe if she finds that she is up against an insensitive,
selfish person who understands nothing less.

One girl may act indignant because she is inexperienced
and has really been taken by surprise by a boy's advances.
Another girl may act indignant if she was too primly
brought up to be able to admit her own sexuality and must
pretend that sex is a repulsive thing which crops up only in
certain males. This was a very common reaction in the
Victorian age, but it is uncommon today.

The experienced girl or woman who is comfortable with
her own feelings and who has learned how easy it is to control the advances of nine out of ten males feels no need to
get angry at the person whose advances she doesn't wel-
come or to make him ashamed. She lets him down graci-
ously by murmuring, for example, 'I'm sorry', as if it were
her fault that a misunderstanding had occurred, or by
promptly laying a restraining hand on his and putting it
back in his territory.

It's common for the boy to try again, right away or later.
He hopes that the girl was just pretending to be reluctant,
so as not to seem too easy. He thinks she is perhaps wanting
and expecting him to persist and that she will look down on
him as a mouse if he doesn't. Her cue is to be as definite at
the second try as she was at the first. But she can still be
friendly, as if appreciating his attention.

Another common manoeuvre of the male is to begin
arguing: 'But you said you liked me.... What's the
harm?... Don't you have any feelings?... Isn't it abnormal not to want to?... All the other girls do.... I don't

want to date a person who doesn't like this side of me.... A boy has strong instincts that have to be satisfied....' There are thousands of arguments that have been used since Adam's time by which the male tries to put the female on the defensive, tries to make her feel she is obliged to explain her 'peculiarity'. There's no point in arguing. Romance and sex are matters of emotions and ideals, not of reasons. From a psychological point of view it is much more persuasive when a girl declines to give reasons, just acts as if she is sure and then changes the subject; for if she can easily be drawn into an argument, it means that underneath she is not at all certain she is right.

A boy who is trying persuade a girl to let him take more liberties than she wants to permit may say frankly that he is not interested in dating a girl who will not give him these pleasures. Or a girl may tell her mother that she must give in to boys, in order to have dates and be popular.

If a girl is reluctant to pet with a boy who mainly wants to use her for his own pleasure, she should tell him to run along. Why should she give away the intimacy that she wants to save for someone she really loves, why should she sacrifice even a small fragment of self-respect, just to be popular with someone of limited appeal? That's a poor bargain. A girl is mistaken who says that 'all the boys' insist on exploiting girls and that a girl will be totally neglected if she doesn't give in. It's true enough that all boys have some desire to pet for petting's sake. But many of them in the early teen years are not ready even to try. Others will not do so because of ideals and inhibitions, even when offered the opportunity. To put this more positively, there are just as many boys looking for a girl to respect and idealise as there are girls looking for such boys. I mean that parents who instil ideals in their children have just as many boys as girls. A girl can be sure that any boy who is drawn to her and who's worth thinking about seriously, far from being angered or disappointed by her unwillingness to pet on slight acquaintance, thinks more of her and wants to know her better.

Of course one reason why a girl may allow herself to be persuaded to give in to loveless petting is that, though part of her wants to save intimacy for a boy she is sure she loves, another conflicting part has physical desire and the urge to experiment and experience—just as the boy does. So she is tempted to use a boy's threats to go away as a cover for her own desires.

Another reason—let's face it—why a girl may give in to a boy who is bold and masterful but who only wants petting is that many of the boys with high ideals are hopelessly bashful and awkward in adolescence. Of course many of the girls with high ideals are shy and awkward in adolescence, too. Most of the bashful girls and the bashful boys improve greatly in charm as they get a little older.

What about the insensitive boy who persists in making advances—even forcibly—despite a girl's sincere resistance? She has to be ready to fight and scream if necessary. But this possibility raises the question whether a girl really has to get into a situation in which she is at the mercy of a boy whose crudeness she was not aware of. The answer generally is no. A girl who isn't looking for trouble doesn't go on dates with or accept rides from boys she doesn't know or knows only slightly. ('No, thanks. Someone else is coming for me.') If she does accept a ride home at night with a boy she knows fairly well and he starts to take a roundabout route, she can immediately explain that she is late already and that they must go by the shortest route. With a boy she knows only fairly well, she shouldn't go on a date that will take them away from other people—not until she has come to know him well and trusts his respect for her. The reason there are stuffy conventions about not accepting rides and dates is to keep girls from getting into unpleasant situations, and a girl shouldn't begin to brush these conventions aside until she's had a lot of experience. Another way to put it is that boys and men on the prowl take it for granted that a girl who accepts rides from semi-strangers is probably looking for excitement. Another way still is to admit that most girls who are 'good' are secretly fascinated with the possibility of being 'bad'. They need to recognise this side of themselves and to keep it under reasonable control, in order to avoid getting into deeper trouble than they really wish.

I don't want to emphasise the exploitive side of males so much that girls will think of all of them with fear or distaste. A great majority of boys and men have been brought up well enough so that a girl can learn to deal with them with confidence and pleasure. This means she must remember that the male is designed to be intrusive and to have to prove his boldness up to the limit she sets. She has to know and to show what the limit is. If he weren't as bold as that limit permits, she'd find him disappointingly tame.

Some of you may want to hear suggestions for guidelines, not to be bound by but to consider. Many young people will call what I suggest too strict or puritanical for themselves. I wouldn't argue—standards and tastes vary widely. Some of you who will like these ideas or ideals as you read them now will find later that you don't always stick to them. This wouldn't be surprising either; it wouldn't mean that the suggestions had not been helpful as ideals. (I didn't always conform to them myself.)

I've suggested that it is preferable for teenagers not to go on individual dates until they are sixteen or seventeen. Even then it's better for them not to spend time petting in secluded places until they have known each other for a year and are confident that a tender, generous love is developing.

I think it's sensible for a teenager not to go beyond kissing and embracing the person he loves until there is some kind of commitment to marriage, which should preferably take another twelve months—two years of knowing each other well and a minimal age of eighteen years. The touching of breasts and genitals even through the clothes is much more exciting and is likely to carry you beyond the point where you can use judgment.

If I say that this conservative advice is based on tragic cases encountered in medical practice, you may be irritated again at the way older people fall back, in their arguments, on greater experience.

Group Companionship

I myself think that the teen years up to sixteen, seventeen or eighteen are generally the time for an informal kind of companionship between boys and girls, mainly in groups.

You get lots of opportunities to learn about the opposite sex and your own sex by being with other young people regularly in school, in Sunday School, in camps, around the neighbourhood, in dropping in and out of other families' homes. This kind of sociability allows you to get to know others casually, which is the most comfortable way for most early adolescents. You can talk as much or as little as you feel like doing, instead of having to fill up all the silences, the way you feel you have to do when there are only two people present. You can be on school and youth club committees to carry out projects and social activities. You can participate in the activity clubs that exist in many schools—a Spanish club, a stamp collectors' club, a nature-study club, etc. There may be plays at school or at a local club or society to act in. There are school and neighbour-hood games to play in, sports events to watch, picnics to go on. There are dances at some schools, at clubs and at homes. In Britain there are many clubs for young people and there are also organisations which foster voluntary service to the community. Many religious organisations sponsor youth clubs, while others are provided by local education authorities or national organisations like the Scout and Guide movements, the Young Farmers' clubs and others. In addition organisations like the Youth Hostels Association, Ramblers' Association, Naturalists' Trust and many sports clubs provide opportunities for young people to take part in activities, either singly or in groups.

Another way to organise social life at this age is of course by group dates—when a crowd goes to the movies, to a bowling alley, to a swimming pool, or the beach, together. These excursions need a parent along in early adolescence, to give leadership, to drive the car, to be sure that a wild character in the group who is trying to prove his courage doesn't get everyone into trouble.

Group activities of all kinds give you opportunities to watch closely other young people of both sexes, see different personalities at work, learn what in the opposite sex appeals to you, learn what members of the opposite sex appreciate or despise, learn what are useful conversational approaches and responses, learn how to let your own good qualities show without having to show off. Those who are most sophisticated, self-assured and talkative naturally take the leadership. The quieter ones can observe and go at their own speed.

When a teenage group gathers in someone's home for a committee meeting, a formal or informal party or a casual get-together, one or two parents should be in the house.

They don't have to be in the same room with the young people or in sight all evening. But they should greet the guests on arrival and the guests should say goodbye to them at the end. They can, for instance, be in the living-room as the guests arrive and then retire to a den or bedroom. Or the guests might go to a recreation room. It is appropriate for parents to drop in with food and drinks or if the party is getting too raucous or too silent. The host-parents have an obligation to the parents of the guests to be near by and to be in charge. All of this is ordinary social courtesy.

Though I think that most teenagers are not ready to appreciate the real values of dating and going steady before they are sixteen or seventeen or eighteen years old (and some not till they are considerably older still), I don't mean that a boy and girl under that age can't ever have a private conversation, away from the crowd. A boy can walk a girl home from school and from other gatherings and parties. He can visit her occasionally at her home (when the family is near by) or even take her to a movie once in a while if her parents know him and approve. What I'd advise against as a regular pattern for young teenagers is weekly, prolonged, secluded dates because they invite progressive physical intimacy before there is real love and because a premature pairing-off takes young adolescents out of circulation just when it is most valuable for them to be finding out about all kinds of young people.

If a young teenage boy should ask a girl to go steady with him, I think she'd be wiser to answer that she appreciates the honour and is fond of him (if she is), but she doesn't think it's sensible to pair off because it's so important at this age to get to know many kinds of people.

Romance and Sex in Later Adolescence

In the later teens—at seventeen, eighteen, nineteen—a majority of young people will have lost enough of their shyness and gained enough experience so that they can mix socially with pleasure. Those who are in love will be in love on a more realistic basis than when they were younger—in the sense that they will have got to know the beloved before allowing themselves to become infatuated, and in the sense that they are seeing each other fairly regularly in real life situations, not just dreaming of each other at a distance. Others will not be emotionally ready yet to fall seriously in love, but they are drawn to certain members of the opposite sex and are having regular or occasional dates.

Aside from the groups just mentioned there will be a fair number of young people remaining who will not feel ready for dating. Some of them will be socially warm and self-assured towards the opposite sex as well as towards their own—it is only in regard to romance and sex that they are unready. Others will be shy both in ordinary sociability and in romance, though they may be well adjusted and productive in their work. In fact some of the world's most creative people—in the arts and sciences—have been this type of shy, late-blooming young people. Most of them will eventually have successful marriages and social lives as well as careers.

I am listing this variety of patterns to point out that each of them can be normal and natural. Most shy people as well as most sociable people are well adjusted. I certainly don't think that a young person who doesn't feel like dating needs to make dates to prove that he can do so. I don't believe a young person of either sex should encourage himself to have a predominantly physical love affair, either, in order to prove to himself that he can.

Another reason why young people who want to go far with their education should not push themselves to become romantically or sexually involved is that there is a reciprocal relationship—to a degree—between studies and sex. Those who are regularly involved in heavy romances or in physical affairs of a kind which keep them in an excited or turbulent state are more apt to have trouble keeping up with their school work. It's not just that their affairs take up time and cause worries. It's more basic than that. Freud pointed out that when a child at the age of six or seven gives up temporarily his romantic and sexual strivings, the emotional energy that is freed is sublimated into school work and other impersonal interests. In adolescence that transformation will be reversed to a small or great degree from impersonal interests to sex. Heads of schools will tell you that if a pupil is given a sports car, providing him with very direct gratifications through dating and showing off, his school work is likely to suffer.

How then does a married student do well academically? The answer is that it depends on how mature the student is when he gets married. If he is a stable, responsible person with a well-fixed ambition, he can perhaps get married at twenty and not have it interfere with his studies, provided his wife is sensible and level-headed too. On the other hand, if he's a distractable person who hasn't settled on a career yet, and he marries or has an affair with a girl who is still emotionally unsure of herself, he may get promptly into academic trouble.

I want to be sure that I don't leave the impression that any time you fall earnestly in love or decide to go steady (on a romantic or physical attraction basis) you will surely fail your exams or lose your life aspirations or cut yourself off from a creative career. That would be going much too far. There are several reasons why: quite a few of the young people who do get interested in each other do not become involved in intense relationships or in day-to-day dating. A majority of the cases of falling in love in the teens do not last long. Those young people who will be going to work after school are more likely to let themselves fall seriously and permanently in love as the time to leave approaches; they can afford to do so, in the emotional sense, because working at a job does not usually require the same mental self-discipline as studying. A majority of those going on to university are, by comparison, more guarded in their feelings. Yet there is a significant number who do drop out of university; becoming involved in an affair or a turbulent marriage is one of the reasons.

'The Arrangement'
(Young People Living Together without Marriage)

In past times there have always been a small number of young lovers who for economic, educational, family or ideological reasons were not married but lived together more or less secretly. In the 1920s an American domestic relations court judge shocked most people by recommending 'Companionate Marriage', trial marriages without children, as a way of attempting to reduce the number of later divorces that are so hard on the children of the family.

In the recent relaxation of sexual standards, a few of the more independent-minded young men and women who are in the last year or so of university and who are away from home anyway have been living together more or less openly without marriage. Some of their parents don't know about it. Some parents have decided the best thing is to pretend they don't know. Some put up with it reluctantly because they aren't positive that it's a mistake or don't see what to do. Some strongly disapprove. Some accept the arrangement quite tolerantly if they have confidence in the stability of their child.

Studies have shown that most of these young people are responsible, thoughtful, studious types who have got to know each other well and developed a genuine affection before setting up joint housekeeping and that they lead quiet, conscientious lives together, like old married couples. A fairly large proportion of them marry in the end. To put it the other way around, they are not devil-may-care, sex-preoccupied, promiscuous people at all.

How is one to judge such a generally disapproved change in custom? The first answer is that we are obviously in a period of rapid change of many traditions and only time will give a sound answer—whether this 'arrangement' will become accepted as a sensible, responsible way for young people to make trial marriages, or whether, with more experience, it will be found to have too many disadvantages in most cases and will be rejected by society.

In the present transitional stage, young people should not try to find an answer in what other youths think or do but in their own ideals and their parents' standards. If the idea is acceptable to them, it may be a responsible way to enter marriage. If it goes against the young person's conscience or if he knows it would cause deep dismay to his parents, he cannot feel right about it, no matter how many of his friends feel differently.

Falling Out of Love or Being Jilted

The burning out of an infatuation can be a painful matter at any age for the person who is still in love, but it is particularly so for the young teenager who has not yet developed any protection against such hurts. There is an aching, stinging emptiness. There is a loss of face, a loss of a sense of dignity, with friends and family. There may be a scalding jealousy if the romance has been ended by the beloved's turning his affection to someone else. There may be a sense of disappointment or indignation or outrage against the erstwhile beloved who now seems a fraud. However, it isn't strictly fair to blame a person for not being able to be what you had imagined him to be.

The pain in the two individuals is usually quite unequal in the break-up, partly because the infatuation was so often unequal from the beginning. (A cynical philosopher once said that a love affair consists of one person who loves and another person who consents to be loved.) In any case, one person is likely to fall out of love long before the other.

Almost all people have gone through these despairs, most often in the early teens. As a result of them, each person becomes a bit more cautious about falling in love again. In the long run this will be helpful to him as long as he doesn't become bitter. Each disappointment helps to educate an individual in how better to find out what other people are really like, how better to know what he himself needs in a beloved. If a person is able to be honest, he may learn what faults of his own contributed to the break-up.

It is wise for the person who has been hurt by love not to make a dramatic show of his wound nor to prolong his suffering. I mean that an individual who has been severely disappointed or angered by what seems like the faithlessness of another may, without quite realising what he is doing, keep telling his friends how badly he has been treated, hoping to be comforted by evoking their sympathy for him and their indignation against the traitor. One trouble with this way of taking it is that it keeps the disappointed lover from getting back on an even keel; he comes to enjoy self-pity. Another is that it's apt to exhaust the patience of his friends. You have to try to act like a good sport, no matter how you feel; let bygones be bygones, chalk it all up to experience, wait for the wound to heal. But if you have deep feelings, the healing will take time.

Since young people are apt to fall in love and fall out of love with more violence and more suddenness than older people, anything that can be done to save heartaches will be valuable. The only plea I can offer is that young people try to be honest with each other if and just as soon as their feelings change. Usually one person begins to have doubts while the other is still passionately in love; the first is then reluctant to say what he feels because he shrinks from admitting that all his vows were mistaken. He hates to cause anguish to his partner and he dreads the arguments and the reproaches. But of course the longer the pretence is kept up, the more painful the relationship becomes for both. So try to be honest at an early stage. Frankness does not mean brutality, as some people think. It can be fair and gentle.

Though there are usually arguments, they solve nothing. The person who has become disenchanted can only repeat again, in some form, the message, 'I don't feel love for you any more.' It is human for the partner still in love to say angry and provocative things. The unfairness of some of these tempts the other person to be cruel, but he should try to resist this.

The person who is feeling deserted will beg for continued dates in the hope that they will clear up what he presumes is a misunderstanding. The other cannot refuse to have one or two more meetings, to avoid the appearance of running away or refusing to listen. But he should refuse to let the issue be confused by turning these into petting dates. (Some females and many males have a simple faith that a little lovemaking will solve all problems.) And he should refuse to have more and more meetings, for these will only prolong the agony.

Now I must make a large exception. I was not referring to lovers' quarrels. They are very common. They are caused by one lover's resentment towards the other over such everyday offences as selfishness, inconsiderateness, unfairness, ungratefulness, laziness, messiness, irritating mannerisms, flirtatiousness, or siding with a relative who criticises the beloved. The resentful one makes accusations. The other responds with counter-accusations which may or may not have anything to do with the case. Or the other simply implies that he doesn't care what the first person dislikes in him, he has no intention of changing. This in a way is the most shocking thing he could say, since the position of both lovers from the start of the romance has been that each would do anything under the sun if it would please the other.

What happens in a lovers' quarrel is that all the petty irritations which have been accumulating for some time but which have been firmly suppressed come boiling to the surface at one time. The reason there are irritations—aside from the fact that everyone has irritating characteristics—is that the lovers are getting to know each other better and also that they are now being a little less careful about showing only their best features.

Far from indicating a fading love, such quarrels in most cases are actually an expression of love, in that each partner cares intensely how the other behaves towards him. Quarrels are also important steps in the adjustment of two people towards each other. Needless to say, two people cannot be a perfect match to start with. Either by quarrels—or by subtler methods of detection, for not all lovers have to quarrel—each finds out what his own irritating characteristics are and tries to modify them. Or he can't or won't modify them, and his beloved decides to put up with them. Or his beloved realises eventually that there are more liabilities than assets and falls out of love.

What determines in the end whether a romance will strengthen into a good marriage or peter out depends on how many good and how many unfortunate qualities there are in a person *in the eyes of his beloved*, on his willingness to see his own faults, on his capacity to change and grow. When I emphasise the phrase 'in the eyes of his beloved' I mean it. People have tastes that are hard to explain. A girl may be impressed with the stuffy egotism of a boy which most other people consider ridiculous. And a boy, otherwise sensible, will be delighted with a baby-talk tone in his girl's pronunciation which turns other people's stomachs.

If your beloved has fallen out of love with you, remember that there is a very human tendency to counteract any sense of being a failure at love by quickly becoming infatuated with someone else—'on the rebound'. You can easily fool yourself and make a fool of yourself when in such a mood. In a majority of cases, however, there is a feeling of depression and of not trusting love which lasts for weeks.

To Tell or not to Tell

If you are in love and are perhaps talking of marriage, better not let yourself be persuaded to reveal previous love affairs or sexual experiences. Your beloved may say, and it sounds plausible, 'We shouldn't have any secrets from each other.' But most people in love don't want to tell and don't want to hear about previous romances—they were mistakes in one way or another. The person who is eager to tell about his past romances is usually someone who gets unconscious pleasure from making his beloved jealous. And the person who wants to know about his beloved's past has, in most cases, an over-jealous personality: it will only make him resentful and miserable to hear the story.

One possible exception, to my mind, would be the case of a girl who has had an illegitimate baby which the neighbours know about. She might feel (though another girl perhaps would not) that it is better to state this briefly at the time when a boy proposes marriage, rather than have him hear it later from someone else. The girl doesn't have to use a tragic tone, as if this episode will turn her boy-friend away permanently, but in the tone of, 'I should tell you, in case it will make a difference to you.'

It sounds cynical to imply that it is all right to deceive as long as you are sure you won't be found out. I only make the distinction because I believe that some men would feel they had been cheated if not told what the neighbours know, whereas they wouldn't feel cheated if not told about previous romances or affairs which no one knows about but the couple involved.

Similarly I think there are many girls who would feel they had been deceived if a boy proposing did not mention he had fathered an illegitimate child.

Shyness is not a Bad Sign

If you are a shy teenager you particularly crave to be sophisticated and amusing. You want to be masterful if you are a boy or seductive if you are a girl. In your class or group in school there are probably individuals who seem much more worldly, witty, well-dressed and successful than you, and you envy them with secret bitterness.

But you should know that the advantage doesn't always lie where it seems to. The individual who at an early age can make the crowd laugh often turns out to be a bore later on. The suave, good-looking boy who seems able to charm all the girls at fifteen may show by eighteen that he has no real personality and nothing to say. The girl who is the vivacious queen of the group in her early teens may just seem noisy a few years later. I don't mean that everyone who starts at the top in appeal finishes at the bottom and vice versa, but there are plenty of drastic shifts.

A boy or girl may be shy in the early teens because, though he has a lot of individuality and character, he realises he has no skill yet in communicating these, in making them interesting to another person. (It's much more difficult at first to express thoughts than it it is to make chit-chat.) He may be especially awkward in talking with a particular individual of the opposite sex just because he feels strongly attracted.

It's good to remember that if you are drawn to someone and if you are a sincere person, the message of your affection will usually get across, despite any awkwardness. This doesn't guarantee that your love will evoke the other's love, though.

How to be Popular

Popularity with a large group is useful only to the politician who's after votes. What you as an individual can use and need is to be appreciated fondly by a small circle of friends for your particular flavour, whether it's for your generosity or understanding or vivacity or witty tongue. Romantically what you as a teenager need is a chance to get to know and be known by some appropriate members of the opposite sex—a few at a time—in order to reveal your own ideas, to learn to respond to the ideas of others, to let your own qualities of personality come out so that those of the other sex who might cherish them can see them, to find out for yourself what qualities you want and need in a beloved. These things are not at all clear to a young person at first. In order to take advantage of your opportunities to get to know members of the opposite sex, you ought to learn enough easy flirtatiousness to signal interest to them. I don't mean a heavy seductiveness but a sparkle in the eye, a personal smile, a lightly flattering remark, to show that you think the other person is fun. You should acquire enough facility with light talk so that you can pass ten minutes or an hour with another person while you—and he—decide whether or not there are possibilities in this friendship.

How to be popular—even with a few people—is the aching problem at the beginning of the teen years. The answer appears elusive except to a few lucky ones, who seem to draw others to them as flowers draw bees. Don't despair. You may have more appealing qualities than you realise. Many of those who have tough going at first have a lot to offer; but they care so much about their relationships that they get paralysed with self-consciousness at first—until they learn some of the lighter approaches.

One approach that young teenagers fall into instinctively, when two or more are thrown together, is to find something interesting or fun to *do*—whether it's dancing, or playing table-tennis or swimming, or looking up a bird's song or playing records. Doing something gets you off the spot of having to make conversation every second. The talk of even the world's best conversationalist will become laboured and painful if he feels he *has* to talk. (Witness the embarrassment of two famous people when asked to talk and smile for a press photographer.)

I'd say that the most important rule, in any of your human relationships (a rule that's broken much more often than it's followed), is to think of the other person rather than of yourself. Then the kinds of questions you can start with are: Where are you from? School or occupation? Future plans? Hobbies? Other interests? This is enough for a three-hour start. If you find that you two are sympathetic, you can go on from these matter-of-course subjects to others which are nearer to the soul, subjects not so easily talked about ordinarily but more satisfying if you've found someone with whom there is real understanding.

Those first questions I listed could be asked impersonally, the way a form for a driving licence asks you questions. They could be asked aggressively, the way a lawyer in court asks them. But if you are making friends or even just making conversation, you must ask questions with a combination of interest, friendliness and sensitivity. More important than your initial questions is your attentiveness to the answers. To be a good conversationalist means to be listening more than half of the time. You must be listening not only with your ears but with your eyes, which you keep on the speaker's eyes, and with your whole facial expression. When he tells you something he considers amusing you naturally smile—at least faintly. When he speaks of how angry he was, you show your sympathetic indignation.

You have to learn to share an enthusiasm for the speaker's subject whether you ever had any previous interest in it or not. If someone speaks to you of his love for golf, and it happens to be a game you've not only never played but have always looked down on, you should be able, if you have an average amount of amiability and flexibility, to generate a conversational interest in it. You could boldly lead from innocence, confess you've never had a club in your hands and ask what the game is really like—just exactly what its joys and frustrations are—what kind of progress the speaker is making. This should not all be dry as dust to you, just because you've never played. You are drawing out the speaker to see what kind of person he is. You are encouraging him to be a good story-teller. You are trying to enhance your own charm as a conversationalist and human being. Perhaps, who knows, you are launching the great love of your life. If it turns out that this is not it, nevertheless you will eventually be using the charm you are developing now when the great occasion comes. The skilful fisherman uses a bit of chicken feather or even a worm to lure the precious trout. You shouldn't look down on what you consider a dull topic when you are on the search for a fascinating person.

When I give you these stage directions, I don't mean that you can fake your responses, like a ham actor. I mean that to be popular in the best sense you have to be a genuinely sympathetic person. In most cases this can be learned. Of course if you are a thoroughly self-centred individual, you can't ever be a sympathetic person and you can't be popular. Most people have enough outgoingness and sympathy to be excellent conversationalists; but they are too thoughtless to make the effort, or they are too self-conscious to let go.

Another similar avenue to popularity is to be willing to share activities. Even if you previously had a dim view of bird watching or carol singing, you can show that you are a good sport and a warm person by being glad to participate because you want to be with the people who are participating.

Some teenagers are capable of sharing an interest or activity, and yet feel so shy about showing their own feelings or responding personally to a companion that they leave him with the impression that they have no warmth at all. The best way to overcome shyness is by taking all opportunities to be with company.

You can also boost your popularity a little by providing good times for your friends: meals, picnics, dancing parties at home or at a club, excursions to other cities. These treats won't do you much good if you are a basically disagreeable or irritating person. But if you have charms that are not easy to see, these shared experiences will give acquaintances the opportunity to appreciate them. By providing good times for others you show your thoughtful side. You give yourself practice in sociability. And, to be materialistic— which is all right as long as you have other qualities too—when others accept your invitations, it puts them under obligation to entertain you in return. Of course a shy teenager may be uneasy about extending such invitations, fearing that they are not conventional in his crowd. Better to take a chance. If you don't dare, let your parents extend the invitations.

Here are a few more small points on popularity or unpopularity.

Quite a few teenagers express their anxiety about being accepted socially or romantically by talking too much, kidding too much or laughing too much. These mannerisms can be very irritating. When in doubt, make too little noise.

You'll never lose the interest of a worthwhile person by quietness. The quiet person is always more intriguing.

If the other person is drawing you out in conversation, don't get so lost in talking about yourself that you forget to stop and turn the conversation the other way.

If you're a girl dealing with a bashful boy, show your interest in only the most gentle ways. Most males are put off by a female who is more aggressive or more seductive than they; this is particularly true of the shy ones.

If you are critical by nature, adolescence will probably accentuate this. Without realising it, you may become so sour or so obsessed with some injustice in the world that you become a bore to most people. Don't give up your critical faculty, but don't harp on your pet indignation when with those who hold an opposite view. Make a point of listening thoughtfully to an opponent and show that you understand his point. It's very easy, too, in adolescence to become hipped on a particular noncontroversial topic or hobby, or to use the same adjective or exclamation to express all strongly felt views. Avoid these handicaps if you become aware of them.

Practice once a day being disarmingly pleasant to one person. It's like putting on a disguise; it's a valuable skill for anyone, whatever his views or purpose.

Dress

Protection is usually mentioned as the first purpose of clothes. Modesty is another, but there is little stress on it today. An aim with high priority throughout history has been to conceal or minimise the unattractive features of each person's body and to call attention to the more appealing ones. When we want to please someone or a group we dress up; and when we don't give a damn or want to show a subtle scorn, we dress too negligently for the occasion.

Human beings have a wavering attitude in regard to modesty and exhibitionism. (Exhibitionism is the pleasurable impulse to show one's body—or one's total self.) They start off in early childhood as frank exhibitionists; they'll gleefully show their navels or their genitals to anyone who really appeals to them. But by six or seven, they are apt to be bashful about being seen naked or when using the bathroom, at least some of the time. In early adolescence, when a person is made strongly aware of his sexual interests but has not yet become sufficiently used to them to be comfortable with them, modesty tends to be even more accentuated. (A modest person may, at the same time, be having fantasies of exhibitionism.)

From mid-adolescence onwards, modesty and exhibitionism are more important issues for the girl than for the boy. Each girl learns to be modest enough to conform—more or less—to the customs of the society or group in which she lives; but she also learns how to make a discreet exhibitionistic appeal to the boys at the same time. It is interesting to realise how the customs vary not only between different groups but with the time of day and the activity. In the daytime, at school or work, the shape of the breasts can be revealed by the cut of the clothes, but the skin of the breasts must not be shown. In a formal evening gown the skin of 49 per cent of the breast can be shown but not the nipple area. At the beach the thigh has been revealed right up to the groin for many years, but until the advent of the miniskirt, this amount of exposure would have been shocking when people were away from the water's edge.

Many girls assume, particularly in these days of relative nudity, that the more skin they reveal, the more attractive

105

they are to the opposite sex. The answer is not this simple. In fact, in a nudist camp or nudist family, the excitement of males at seeing female bodies is, relatively speaking, at a low ebb. (I'm not saying it is absent.) In a striptease show, the performer knows that she would be a failure if she took off her clothes in her dressing-room, stalked out on to the stage and stood there. One aspect of the success of the show is the gradualness of the revelations. The spectators are constantly keyed up by the hope and expectation of more to come. Most exciting is the artful way in which the stripper keeps moving about, starts to take off a garment, hesitates, delays, slips it off, but then, quicker than the eye can see, drapes it or holds it in front of her so that much less is revealed at that moment than had been expected. Her reluctance (fake though it is) is what imparts value to her eventual revelations. To the man in the audience it is as if he is trying to persuade her to disrobe and she is hesitantly yielding. Her performance permits him to imagine that he is the active person.

(Similarly in dating. It is the basic nature of the male to be the pursuer. The seeming uncertainty of the girl—about whether she likes him or whether she will allow him to make any advances—is what excites him and spurs him on. When a girl on a date acts more 'forward' than the boy, her aggressiveness, in most cases, lessens his enthusiasm and initiative.)

You can see why clothes that half conceal are more provocative than clothes—or lack of clothes—that only reveal.

Exhibitionism is all relative. In Victorian times a man would be excited, according to the novels, to catch a glimpse of a girl's ankle as she climbed into a carriage or bus—more excited, I suspect, than today's man who has seen much of a girl's thigh in a comparable situation.

Perhaps all that I'm expressing here is a prejudice against

the homeliness and anticlimax of most nudity. I know well from doing thousands of physical examinations as well as from what I see at the beach that few individuals are so well formed that they look beautiful when naked or near-naked. Ninety-five out of a hundred people are much improved by clothes.

Styles in clothes change faster than other styles, especially for women, not only in such obvious respects as whether hems and waistlines go up or down, but also as to whether a woman is to look childish or sophisticated, feminine or gladiatorial.

Adolescents and youths in Western nations have usually had their own styles in clothes, as they have their own styles in entertainers, music, vocabulary and so on. Partly this is because during their long years of schooling and training, they are not accepted into adult society as fully participating members, the way teenagers are in many simpler societies. Not being accepted, they emphasise their separateness. Partly it is because their basic rebelliousness makes them prefer to be quite different from their parents and their parents' generation, in all their tastes and standards.

The intensity of the revolt of youth, beginning in the late 1960s, which has expressed itself in such matters as the assertion of a freer and franker sexual code, in the rejection of competitiveness and materialism as the most admirable virtues, in a new recognition of the saving grace of love in all its forms, has also stimulated in some individuals a preference for clothes that are either severely plain or rumpled, and also for an ungroomed appearance. They decline to make the effort to look pleasing to others or to themselves. This attitude has elements of defiance, of self-denial, of pride in being able to do without, of independence even from one's own age group. I admire the courage, independence and idealism that these people show. But I am always hoping that they will find other, more constructive ways of expressing these qualities, and can then revert to an attractive appearance.

I'm not decreeing that one type of dress or grooming is better than another just because I like it. Styles must swing—from formal to informal and back again, and from colourful to sombre. What I have been regretting is deliberate dinginess and messiness, which is not really a matter of style but of nose-thumbing—no matter how idealistic the nose-thumber is in other respects.

[III]

Love, Pseudo-Love and
Sexual Deviations

Varieties of Love

There are at least half a dozen quite different varieties of love, all of which go by the same label. In infancy and early childhood love is principally dependent: the small child is tied tightly to his mother, turns to her for all his wants, feels anxious if she is away for long, is elated when she returns. Though dependent love decreases throughout childhood, there is, of course, still an attachment to parents in adulthood. Even married love has a dependent element in it. Love of God is, in part, like the dependent love of parents, though it usually has other spiritual and mystical qualities as well.

By about the age of three, a child begins to be able to love other children companionably and generously, loves his parent of the same sex with intense admiration and develops a romantic and sexual and possessive love for the other parent. These all come under the heading of spontaneous, outgoing love.

You love a good friend because of easy, frank communication, a similar sense of humour, interests in common, his loyalty to you, his need of you, his approval of you.

In adulthood a mature sexual–romantic love is a fusion of two very dissimilar emotions. One is physical, crude, relatively undiscriminating. The other is generous, tender, idealistic. An amazing combination.

We all love ourselves to one degree or another in the sense of thinking of ourselves a lot, wanting others to admire us, being eager to talk about ourselves to a good listener. But some of us can disguise our self-love more successfully and therefore are less boring about it. One of the biggest differences in human beings is between those who love only themselves and those who love others more.

Emotions Masquerading as Love

Many feelings aside from the conventional ones go to make up love relationships. I'll mention some cases I've seen personally.

A younger sister becomes engaged and marries. Her older sister suddenly discovers that she does love the boy who has been hanging around for a couple of years and who, she always said before, was just a nuisance. Rivalry with her sister may have made her exaggerate her love for the person who was available. On the other hand, it's also possible that in her deeper feelings she has been in love with the boy for some time, but that for complicated psychological reasons she wasn't ready to recognise these feelings. She covered them up by telling everyone, including herself, that she disliked him; then suddenly the awareness of love broke through the denial, with full force. This is actually a fairly common pattern for falling in love, in boys as well as girls.

An attractive but selfish man who is popular with girls and presumably could have his pick appears to fall in love with and marries a rather plain, uncharming girl who is wealthy. Whether or not it had an influence in this case, wealth is one charm in a person which does not become boring with time or wither with age.

A man marries a colourless girl who finds him fascinating. Devotion and admiration from a spouse can make up for the absence of many other virtues.

A girl who has always felt that her family was socially

inferior when compared with the neighbours falls in love with a dull young man whose family is top drawer. This does not imply cynicism or materialism on her part. His position is truly lovable to her.

A good-looking young hussy resolves to snare a sixty-year-old widower with a large fortune. Her charms of body and manner infatuate him utterly and he marries her. He tells his friends that he loves her for her warmth, her sincerity and her devotion to him, but his friends are quite sceptical about these virtues. Still, if she continues to give him sufficient attention, his wishful thinking, his sexuality and his pride will do the rest.

Boys and men like to imagine that the female who has the most revealing clothes or seductive manner is the one with the highest sexual responsiveness. Usually this is far from the truth. The dramatically seductive female is sometimes quite hostile towards men and is dangling her charms with the unconscious aim of snaring men rather than pleasing them or loving them.

An attractive, sought-after girl who has been antagonistic to her very conventional parents for a long time falls in love with and marries a man from a minority group against which her parents have a violent prejudice. This doesn't mean that she doesn't love him for truly attractive qualities; but still one of the most appealing and exciting things about him *may* be her parents' wish to forbid the match. While we are on this topic I'd like to add some unsolicited advice. I think it is wonderful that so many young people now are unprejudiced and are helping to fight prejudice. I hope that some day race, religion and ethnic background can be ignored by lovers (as well as by employers and landlords and neighbours). But where prejudices are strong, I think young people should be extra-cautious in marrying across such barriers. Marriage is a difficult adjustment for most couples even when all the conditions seem favourable. Barriers of prejudice often add intolerable strains. They may come from families and friends on both sides. To use marriage to show lack of prejudice or to fight prejudice is like trying to pry a huge boulder with a thin stick. The boulder doesn't get moved, but the stick does get broken. I'm not saying that marriage across barriers can't succeed, but that it takes superhuman love and maturity to make it succeed. If you are considering it, have a long engagement, to make sure.

Attraction only to 'Bad' Girls

There are boys who can feel no physical attraction to a girl they respect or have tender feelings for—they respond only to 'bad' girls or girls who would be considered entirely unsuitable by their parents. This disturbance is fairly common—for girls as well as boys—in the early years of adolescence, but tends to wear off in a majority of cases. In a few unfortunate individuals it persists for life. (A persistent case may yield to psychiatric treatment.)

The disturbance is caused by an excessive inhibition of sexuality in the six- to eight-year-old period, when the boy comes to feel a taboo that is particularly strong against any romantic interest in his mother, for whom his respect and tenderness are the highest. Next in order come his sisters and other 'nice' girls close to the family. And if, as in most such cases, he has grown up with an unusually strong feeling that sex is a dirty business, this makes it doubly sinful to associate it with good girls or women. All the sexual drive he allows himself to recognise is then channelled towards debased members of the opposite sex. Girls with the corresponding problem can feel no sexual response to men for whom they feel respect and tenderness.

The Lechery of Males

The fact that physical sexuality is generally more insistent in the male and is less tightly tied to the tender, romantic and spiritual side of love than in the female means that carefully brought-up girls may be shocked at one time or another by the crude behaviour of males—even those males who have high standards in other respects.

The boy who, on a date, suddenly makes advances to you without any warning or encouragement has been discussed earlier. He's either inexperienced and unsure of himself or he's a crude self-centred person who thinks only of his own pleasure.

You may be more startled some day to have a respectable older man—even the father of a good friend—make advances to you. He is being carried away by an infatuation that has overcome his good judgment. It's a compliment of sorts. If he's thinking at all, he's hoping that you're secretly fond of him and that you'll enjoy or at least won't mind his indiscretion. Your cue is promptly to make it very clear that you don't feel that way about him and that he must stop. Usually the respectable man who acts so rashly is quickly cooled by this kind of refusal. It is apt to frighten him into a realisation that he may be gossiped about all over town or that the girl's father might even bring him into court. The girl in these situations usually doesn't need to scream or fight, as long as she is quite definite. But if she is half intrigued, only half indignant, the man will persist.

Scalp Collectors

There is a kind of boy or man who appears to have a great romantic interest in a girl, but who, as soon as she falls in love with him, loses interest. His special pleasure is in persuading a girl to love him; but he has no use for her love and may be heartless in abandoning her. He'll be quick to seek another girl's love. He is sometimes called a scalp collector. This pattern may sometimes be traced through psychoanalysis all the way back to the small boy's frustrated yearning to win his mother for himself and his resentment at her for not responding as he wished. He's unconsciously taking revenge on his girl-friends for what he considered, at five, his mother's heartlessness. He's usually an immature, self-centred person in addition. A girl or woman may be a scalp collector too.

Another pattern which is also related to the small child's frustrated romantic yearning for his parent is that of the person of either sex who is always hopelessly in love with someone who doesn't return the feeling, but is invariably uninterested in those who are romantically drawn to him.

Possessiveness and Jealousy

Some people are highly possessive in their love relationships, others hardly at all. Some enjoy being possessed; others hate it and struggle to get free.

Closely related but not quite the same thing is jealousy. There are lovers and spouses who will become jealous on the slightest provocation; and some of the people who are loved this way are pleased to be guarded so closely. Others realise that they cannot stand the confinement, and that the relationship must be given up to avoid endless misery.

There is another kind of individual, fairly common, male or female, who enjoys—unconsciously—making his beloved jealous; for him this is part of the pleasure of a love relationship. In most cases he doesn't realise what he's doing. Frequently he had a possessive, jealous parent of the opposite sex and learned unconsciously to tease the parent in this particular way from a young age. As an adult he may be attracted to and marry a possessive, jealous type; then the stage is set for an endless continuation of the same jealousy-provoking pattern.

Sexual Deviations

By the time an ordinary human being is emotionally mature, his strongest love relationship will be with his spouse, and the climax of his sexual activity and pleasure will be sexual intercourse.

When the emotional development of the child does not progress according to the regular scheme, we can see deviations in the end results.

There are various body zones and various means by which a human being gains sensual pleasure. The infant uses his mouth for his two enormously important joys—eating and sucking. By the age of three or four years children have the instinct to become involved occasionally in sex play with themselves and with each other, which may include touching, looking at each other's anatomies, showing themselves. They also peep at their parents when they get a chance.

In adulthood these and other childhood means of gaining sensual pleasure still have strong appeal, as is shown by

116

men and women kissing and fondling, by men's going to striptease shows and buying naked-girlie magazines, by women wearing revealing evening dresses and bathing suits. But by this age these mouth, touching, looking, revealing pleasures are usually subordinate and preliminary steps in lovemaking which lead up to intercourse.

A sexual activity is often called deviant if some other pleasure than intercourse is its chief aim, or if it is carried out between two people who are not of opposite sexes or if one partner is only a child. A few deviations are definitely harmful in that one person takes advantage of another—an adult seducing a child, a strong person inflicting a cruel or offensive act on an unwilling victim. On the other hand, most deviations are only slightly off the usual track and both partners participate willingly.

Homosexuality

Homosexuality is a sexual love for a person of the same sex. ('Homo' means 'same'.) A person is called an overt homosexual if he has been involved in an actual affair or at least is consciously aware of his desires. On the other hand a psychiatrist may refer to a person as a latent homosexual if he believes—from the individual's behaviour or thought processes—that there is a strong homosexual disposition in the unconscious part of his mind, of which he himself has no conscious awareness.

There are really two aspects to homosexuality as the term is commonly used. In the first a person identifies with, feels and acts like, a person of the opposite sex—the effeminate man or the masculine woman. This person may or may not be aware of homosexual desire. In the second a person's sexual desire goes predominantly towards a person of the

117

same sex; in other respects he may appear and act like a normal person, or he may show the first (identification) aspect too.

You can't say simply that one individual is a homosexual and another is not. It's a relative matter. All people of both sexes have at least a bit of homosexuality in the sense that they can identify to one degree or another with those of the opposite sex—sensing intuitively how they feel. If males couldn't identify at all with females, and vice versa, they wouldn't have enough sensitivity to each other's emotions to be able to live compatibly together as man and wife.

The normal bisexuality of males and females becomes apparent in another way. Many adults who are considered normal, especially males, would, if deprived of the company of the opposite sex for months at a time, and if they hadn't been taught that this was immoral and shameful, become aware of some physical attraction to members of their own sex. Homosexual activity on this basis has been fairly common among prisoners and among sailors on long cruises.

Normal homosexuality shows up in another way during the years of puberty development and early adolescence, in the tendency of quite a few young people to first feel a strong attraction and admiration for a grown-up or a youth of the same sex as himself. This is explained primarily on the basis that the taboo against interest in the opposite sex, which was so intense from about six to eleven years, can't be outgrown in a hurry.

The Kinsey Reports indicated that a fair percentage of boys (fewer girls) have some homosexual experiences during adolescence.

Some of those whose desire is predominantly homosexual also have some responsiveness to the opposite sex.

The non-effeminate male homosexual may appear, in

manner and interests, no different from the average normal man. But for deeply unconscious reasons (often having their main roots in the small boy's anxious misunderstanding about why girls are made different from boys) he can't feel physically responsive to a person who has no penis. That is to say, a woman's lack of penis stirs up so much anxiety in his unconscious mind that it obliterates sexual desire. In a compensatory way he tends to be drawn to boys and young men whose fineness of skin and softness of flesh seem relatively feminine. In other words, he likes women except for their lack of penis, and when he turns to a boy or man to love instead, he wants him to seem as much like a woman as possible.

Men and boys who are effeminate tend to feel like women, to have interests like women's, to speak and have the mannerisms of women. Some of them in private dress like women. They often get along unusually well with women in the sense of companionableness. But they want to be loved—physically and emotionally—by another man, as a woman is loved by a man.

Psychiatrists believe that one factor in early childhood which commonly pushes a boy towards an effeminate and homosexual disposition is having grown up with a father who was unusually distant and uncomfortable with him or a father who was the non-dominant partner in his parents' marriage. This left the boy with an exaggerated need to be accepted by a man. It also deprived him of an impressive masculine model to pattern himself after; for to want to grow up to be like a person one must have felt loved and accepted by him.

Another factor common in the background of the effeminate male homosexual is having had a mother who was excessively wrapped up in her son and overly possessive towards him, a mother who drew him to herself by confiding in him and sharing all her feminine interests with him. In this way he acquired a stronger-than-average identification with a woman. You might say, to oversimplify, that his father pushed him away from masculinity and his mother pulled him towards femininity.

There is often not as sharp a line as I've implied between effeminate and non-effeminate male homosexuals. The great majority are effeminate to a greater or lesser degree. Though many homosexuals are unhappy—in part because they feel scorned and persecuted—and all feel great emotional need for strong homosexual relationships, these relationships in fact are often frustratingly brief and beset with jealousies, and of course they also lack the satisfactions of parenthood.

In some countries such as Britain the law permits homosexual acts in private between consenting adults over twenty-one. But the laws of most Western nations consider homosexual acts to be crimes, even between consenting adults, and the police regularly harass suspects. There is a movement among homosexuals to get such laws repealed on the basis that what adults prefer to do in private is only their own concern. Psychiatrists believe that the unconscious reason why societies have made such harsh laws against acts that harm no one is people's fear of their own unrecognised perverse impulses, as well as the primitive but important need for society to breed.

When a boy or adolescent is approached by a strange man who suggests going to his room on one excuse or another, the boy usually only needs to be very definite in saying no to discourage the man.

A girl may acquire a masculine identification if she grows up as her father's intensely close companion and confidante. This identification is particularly apt to occur if there has also been an unusually strained relationship between the girl and her mother (there is normally always a little strain), so that she has never looked forward pleasurably to becoming a woman, like her mother. Feeling more like a man, she picks up masculine mannerisms and interests. Her sexual interest, consciously or unconsciously, may then turn predominantly to women. If she becomes an overt homosexual, she has a desire to be the active person in seeking a partner and in making love by some kind of physical stimulation.

There are other women homosexuals who are quite feminine in appearance and attitude but who want to be loved passively by a woman more than by a man. Love-making by a man may be repugnant to them because of early childhood impressions and interpretations. In many cases there is a combination of these two tendencies, and the degree of obvious masculinity varies greatly.

Sadism and Masochism

The Marquis de Sade, after whom sadism is named, got his principal sexual pleasure from inflicting physical pain on women. (They were willing—in fact, eager—victims.) But the term is usually used in a much broader sense than that. The sadist may inflict mental as well as physical suffering. He may be sadistic mainly towards a person with whom he is in love or he may be sadistic towards almost everyone he deals with. There are women sadists too. The sadist was made like that by growing up in a family in which there was above-average cruelty somewhere.

The masochist enjoys suffering. There are dramatic stories about the uncommon individuals who crave to be whipped, for instance, as a regular part of their sexual pattern. Such a pattern may go way back to early experiences in which a child was caught in sex play and severely pun-

121

ished; thus sexual excitement and punishment got linked together.

But in a less dramatic way the enjoyment of suffering enters into many relationships which are not considered sexual in the ordinary sense, and the pain may be entirely mental. There are married couples who fight constantly, some by hurling crockery, others by hurling insults. In one case the wife irritates and taunts her husband until he attacks; in another they take turns provoking each other to violence. New neighbours, hearing the curses and screams, assume that the marriage is breaking up; but such a marriage can go on for a lifetime. In other words, a man and woman, no matter how much they complain about each other, may really need this kind of relationship. If they ever did get divorced they'd have to find new spouses equally quarrelsome. In some such couples there is a close connection between their fights and their sexuality; they typically make love when making up after a quarrel.

Sadism and masochism shouldn't be thought of as essentially perverse. To a degree they are normal aspects of human nature. Ordinary kidding is sado-masochistic. Fishing and hunting for game are in part sadism. When a subordinate in a military or business organisation says 'Yes, sir!' with enthusiasm to a superior who is giving him an order, there is an element of masochism in the submissive gesture. The men who suffer agonies in climbing the Himalayas are able to do so because of masochism.

There may be a more or less normal masochism, as well as a normal aggression, and a desire to prove their potency too, in male youths when they carry out such dangerous acts as driving a car at eighty miles per hour on a dare or trying out a habit-forming drug. As a matter of fact, there are several overlapping factors that contribute to such actions. There is a yearning, as a part of growing up, to experience all sensations. There is the compulsive need, as a new, untried near-adult, to prove one's stamina, daring, stoicism, ability to do without. Quite a few older men will do such things on occasion, especially when put on a spot, but they aren't always looking for chances to take. However, a few men will take any risk right up to old age.

For the person getting into the teen years, the important thing is to be aware of the sado-masochistic aspect of human relations and to avoid getting tangled up with individuals who are too cruel or who bring out the cruelty in you. If you find that this keeps happening despite your wishes, you need psychiatric advice.

Some other Deviations

There are several varieties of somewhat similar sexual be-haviour which occur mainly in adolescent boys who have been brought up in a much more inhibited way than most and with somewhat mixed-up feelings about sex. The youth who is called a Peeping Tom has an intense desire to see a girl undressed, as all other males do to a degree, that may be traced to his having been excessively excited by things he saw when peeping in early childhood. But he is too shy in other respects to try to achieve his desire by getting to know a girl and reaching some stage of intimacy with her. The Peeping Tom may be content to watch a girl's window for hours from within his own house, or he may become so bold as to climb a fire escape or tree on someone else's property, which may result in the police being called. In a great majority of cases a young Peeping Tom is no more dangerous to the girls and women of the neighbourhood than the average boy or man. But since he frightens girls and women with his secretiveness and his trespassing, there are laws against his activities. Another youth who is too inhibited to date any girl he might know at school or in the neighbourhood may try to make a slow, stealthy pass at an unknown girl sitting next to him in a cinema. Even more shy is the youth who cannot make a deliberate approach to a known or unknown girl but seeks opportunities to be crowded close to girls in buses or trains. (If he is too purposeful, he is sometimes called a 'masher' in city slang.)

In most of the cases above, the boy gradually emerges from his strongly inhibited condition and makes in adulthood a sexual and social adjustment within the normal limits. (If he doesn't he should seek psychoanalytic help.) But in youth he needs to be reminded that if a girl or her parents should complain to the police, it might be embarrassing or worse.

I'd like to take this occasion to warn boys who earn money as sitters that a girl in the three- to six-year-old period can become very seductive if for instance she gets excited in rough-housing, just because she is at the early-childhood sexual–romantic stage, yet hardly knows what she's doing. A youth with strong sexual feelings of his own may find it difficult to resist such a disarming temptation to sex play unless he's somewhat prepared. As a matter of fact it's better for older boy sitters to avoid exciting games with young children.

The men who occasionally molest little girls are often (not always) lonely, unsuccessful people, middle-aged or beyond, who have been inadequate in most ways in dealing with adults. A majority do nothing more than fondle, though this is frightening enough to the girl and to the whole neighbourhood. A minority are potentially brutal because of a loveless, cruel upbringing.

The men who are called sex criminals in the newspapers

all sound like fiends. Some are and some aren't. The youths and men who are dangerous to others (and therefore ultimately to themselves) are those who have a strong impulse to get to sexual relations by forcibly overcoming a girl's resistance or, even if she is initially willing, to hurt her in the process. These cruel impulses tied to sex usually come from having been reared from childhood by cruel parents. A young girl doesn't need to fear that friendly boys from her own neighbourhood may turn unexpectedly into fiends. In the first place fiends are rare; and they have unusual personalities, often being without much warmth or humour or openness. The boy who has fantasies (daydreams) about cruel acts should consult a psychiatrist, to see if treatment is called for, in order to avoid the possibility of real tragedy.

Prostitutes are women who make a living by offering themselves sexually to men who will pay. A few are nymphomaniacs (women with an excessive sexual desire). Others are incapable of true love or they are unconsciously out to cheat men by only pretending to love them or they are unconsciously shaming their parents. Some are drug addicts desperate for money. Most grew up without much self-respect.

Obscenity

Obscenity means sexual material in literature or art, or sexual behaviour in movies, on the stage or in public that is considered offensively lewd (whatever the intention of the creator or seller). Pornography is matter designed with the deliberate purpose of causing sexual excitement.

In recent years the courts have excused more and more of what used to be considered objectionable. British law defines as obscene any writing or article that 'tends to deprave and corrupt'. The United States' Supreme Court now calls a production obscene only if it is clearly designed to 'appeal to prurience' and at the same time is 'utterly without redeeming social value'. A recent film story about delinquency showed scenes of brutality, prostitution, homosexuality and sodomy which 'revolted' the judges who saw it; but they called it not obscene because it could be thought of as having educational value.

From my particular point of view, to judge a work only on these two technical grounds misses the main purpose of obscenity laws, which is to protect people from being revolted or brutalised by crude sexual material—or by brutality without sex for that matter. I think the need for this kind of control is particularly important in a country which has sky-high rates of crime and delinquency and which has been endlessly fascinated with violence on television.

I agree that we overdid prudery and propriety in the Victorian period—we tried to deny our sexuality and our aggression altogether, and the insincerity was corrupting. But I myself think we have swung much too far in the opposite direction. It is revealing that the countries which have recently gone the furthest in legalising and indulging in pornography are Sweden, Denmark and the United States, all of which were outstandingly puritannical up to a few decades ago. Though it's natural enough for the people of most countries to have their naughty, half-secret fun by allowing sexuality to come partway out of repression, I believe we are now deliberately coarsening and brutalising sex to prove to ourselves that we are not puritans any more. I feel this is not healthy for our sexual relations or for our idealism or for our civilisation in general.

I believe that children in particular should be protected from being shocked by stumbling on crude literature, pictures, films, plays or TV programmes, because they are in the developmental period when character and ideals are in a sensitive and formative state. It is a somewhat different matter when an older adolescent or youth has become curious enough to want to search out very purposefully, for instance, the pornographic literature that is kept out of sight in the public library, or the pictures he can borrow from a friend or buy under the counter. To find these by his own efforts will not be as disillusioning to a sensitive person as having them displayed before him with the approval of the law. Of course all teenagers worth their salt will claim that they are sophisticated enough to be able to take pornography without upset; but this assertion really comes from curiosity and from the ambition to be grown up rather than from a sure knowledge of being unshockable. I do believe that crude or brutal obscenity is disturbing to young people with high ideals, particularly until the age of eighteen or nineteen, when attitudes are better formed. As a matter of fact it is at least slightly shocking to older people too (including myself) unless they are quite coarse to start with.

[IV]
Adolescent Worries

Self-Consciousness and Fear of Illness

Several factors make an adolescent uncomfortably aware of himself and worried about his physical and mental health: his rapidly changing body draws his attention inwards. So do his turbulent new feelings. A tendency to guiltiness about sex—even in this day of much greater tolerance—often lies behind his vague fears that he may have harmed his body, that he has acquired a venereal or other disease, that he is losing his mind.

Underlying these factors is the uneasy sense of having lost his earlier identity as a child of the family and of not yet having acquired an independent one as an adult.

A teenager because of such worries has a special need of a sympathetic teacher at school or a social worker, or an understanding doctor or clergyman.

Masturbation

In former times, before anything was known scientifically about the psychology or physiology of sex, it was believed that masturbation was harmful physically and mentally: that physically it would cause weakness and impotence; mentally that it would cause various forms of nervousness and even insanity. These beliefs caused much worry in young people. Now we know that they are not true. But this knowledge hasn't solved all the fears about masturbation.

Masturbation is the sexual stimulation of oneself, usually

while having sexual fantasies. It is most commonly done of course by stimulating the penis or the clitoris with the hand. But some individuals, strongly inhibited in childhood against touching the genital, have learned instead how to rub it against bedding or other objects or to squeeze it between the thighs. There is also vaginal stimulation.

Several overlapping reasons are usually given for the almost universal occurrence of masturbation in adolescence in the industrialised countries. Young people have strong sexual urges for some time before they begin to date and even longer before they have intercourse. There usually has to be a prolonged postponement of marriage until they finish their elaborate educations. The ideal of chastity until marriage or engagement, the fear of permanent commitment to the wrong person and the fear of pregnancy have kept many youths with high aspirations from love affairs before marriage. So, masturbation has usually served as a substitute for intercourse. Actually, masturbation has become much less of a worry for young people in the past twenty-five years as sexuality in various forms has been shorn of much of its mystery and guilt, as improved contraceptive methods have reduced the fear of pregnancy for those not concerned about chastity, and as prosperity has made student marriages possible.

The young people who are still most concerned about masturbation are those who grow up in families with high ideals, part of whose sexual interest and energy is sublimated into aspirations and creativity. The sublimation is what enables them to go on for years in their studies, postponing some of the other immediate gratifications, makes them dream of idealised marriages and makes many of them distinctly hesitant—in their own feelings—about becoming involved in casual sexual affairs. For such people, in whom the direct expression of sexuality is partly blocked for years,

131

the impulse to masturbate, with fantasies, is intense and usually irresistible.

Young people ask whether, for sure, masturbation is physically and mentally harmless and the answer is yes. (There is no truth in the statement sometimes heard that masturbation is harmless only if practised in moderation.) But the knowledge that masturbation is not harmful does not take away the worry and guilt altogether. First, a great majority of human beings are so constituted and conditioned that they feel at least slight guilt about any sexuality except in marriage, however enlightened they have become. Secondly, people with strict standards inevitably feel that a solitary form of sexuality which offers no affection to another person is unattractive, even though it may seem less objectionable than intercourse without real love.

According to the Kinsey Reports, people with relatively little in the way of education and aspirations, who on the average come to intercourse earliest in adolescence because they have the least inhibition against it, are more apt to consider masturbation (and other forms of sexuality that are not intercourse) to be immoral and repugnant. So the attitudes are reversed at the upper and lower ends of the educational scale.

Ache in the Groin

A boy who is involved in petting which causes him to have erections for long periods without orgasm is apt to develop an ache which seems to be located vaguely in the lower abdomen or in the groin (the groove between abdomen and thigh) or in the testicles. This ache may last for a day or so at a time. The medical name for the condition is varicocele.

Erection of the penis is brought about partly by a constriction of the veins which lead the blood away from the penis. This same constriction causes an engorgement of the veins coming from the testicles and the seminal vesicles and this is the explanation of the ache in varicocele. In Nature's scheme of things, sexual excitement is expected to lead to intercourse with orgasm, and that puts an end to the constriction of the veins. A boy who is made uncomfortable by this aching yet who desires to continue the petting may be able to solve the problem by allowing or encouraging himself to have an orgasm at such times. This suggestion is made on the assumption that he has been trying all along to hold the orgasm back because he thought it might be embarrassing to have the emission of semen in his clothes. But the amount is really small and though he may be very conscious of this, it is unlikely that it will be noticeable to his girl or anyone else.

Impotence

Sexual impotence is the inability for a boy or man to have an effective erection and ejaculation. (Impotence should be differentiated from infertility—which, in the case of a man, usually means that his sperm have proved incapable of fertilising his wife's ova; on laboratory examination his sperm may be shown to be inactive.) Some impotent men have very little erection and no ejaculation. Others have an inadequate erection and, right away, an ejaculation. (*Ejaculatio praecox* is the Latin term for this, meaning a premature ejaculation, before there is adequate erection for inserting the penis in the vagina.)

There are two types of impotence which are more or less normal. An adolescent boy who has been very strictly brought up in regard to sex and girls may have little or no erection in the first year or so of his dates. Then he may gradually develop a normal potency. At the opposite end of the age scale, most men in their sixties and seventies become progressively more impotent. (There is little lessening of their interest in sex and women.)

A few cases of lifelong impotence are due to physical disease or injury—for instance, a spinal injury with paralysis from the waist down. But the overwhelming majority are psychological in their causation. Psychoanalysis has shown that most of these can be traced back to frightening experiences or the teaching of fearful attitudes towards sexuality in early childhood. Some cases of impotence can be cured by psychoanalysis, which seeks to recall the basis of the child's anxious misunderstandings, so that they can be corrected.

Some men are impotent with most women but potent with just one. They will give up a lot to have that woman. Or they are potent only in very special circumstances.

Most men would rather suffer any other disability than impotence. This is not primarily because of the pleasure missed. It is because the core ambition, pride and satisfaction for most men is to be virile, manly. The meaning is somewhat different for each man but it may take in such aspects as showing competitiveness, courage, pugnacity, having a powerful car, earning and having money—as well as physically satisfying a woman. These aims seem related to each other, in a man's feelings, and sexual impotence threatens them all. (However, some men with lifelong impotence have been extraordinarily productive in their careers and have had generally satisfactory marriages, so impotence is not disastrous in actuality.)

Frigidity

The sexual disturbance in girls and women which roughly corresponds to impotence in males is called frigidity. A frigid woman is unable to feel pleasure in physical contact with men, especially in intercourse. Some of these women find any sexual contact distasteful or repulsive, and intercourse actually painful.

Frigidity can usually be traced to unfortunate experiences or excessively fearful attitudes acquired in early childhood. It can sometimes be cured by psychoanalysis.

There are quite a few girls and young women, especially those brought up with high ideals, who are slow to be aroused sexually and who reach orgasm infrequently or not at all. A great majority of these become progressively more responsive with time or after giving birth to their first child.

[V]
Anatomy and
Physiology of Sex

Prepuberty Growth Spurt

Technically speaking, puberty is the moment when a child reaches sexual maturity. In the girl this is the first menstrual period. In the boy there is no equally dramatic sign. Since this moment comes at the age of twelve in the average girl and fourteen in the average boy, the child is not fully grown and is far from emotional maturity. And, in a society which counts on more and more education, a child of this age is still further away from financial and social independence. As a matter of fact, the first menstrual period does not even represent full physical sexual maturity, because a girl usually cannot become pregnant until a year or so later. Adolescence, technically speaking, is the stage of gradually slowing physical growth and turbulent emotional development which lasts for several years *after* the moment of puberty.

Before puberty there are two to three years of the prepuberty growth spurt. This phase lasts from age ten to twelve in the average girl and from twelve to fourteen in the average boy. A girl who was previously growing in height at the rate of one and a half inches and in weight at five pounds per year suddenly speeds up to about three inches and fifteen to twenty pounds per year. Her breasts begin to develop (one often starts before the other); then her pubic (genital) hair and axillary (armpit) hair appear. After two years of accelerated growth and development, she has acquired a fairly womanly figure, with rounded breasts and broadened hips, and her first period occurs. In the following year she may grow one inch, and in the two years after that probably not more than an inch more altogether. Her figure will continue to become more womanly for several years.

The average boy begins his prepuberty growth spurt at about twelve and increases in height at three or four inches a year and in weight at fifteen to twenty-five pounds a year, for about two years. His penis and testicles enlarge, and his pubic hair and then his axillary and face hair begin to grow. Later his voice changes. By the end of two years he has acquired a fairly manly figure and most of his manly size. However, he will continue to grow at a slower and slower rate for two to three years more, adding a couple more inches altogether.

There are widely different timetables for puberty development. Though the average age for girls to start the growth spurt is ten, there are quite a number who start as early as nine or as late as eleven, a few at eight or twelve and an occasional one at seven or thirteen.

It would be helpful if early developers took *longer* than the usual two years to reach puberty and if late starters could reach it in less than two years, so that everyone could even up. But it works just the opposite way. Early starters sometimes reach puberty in one and a half years, and late starters may take two and a half years. It's also unfortunately true that usually the tallest children get their growth spurt earliest and the short children begin late. So everything conspires to accentuate shortness or tallness during the puberty years.

Patterns of early or later puberty growth tend to run in families. They are rarely due to any abnormality.

Most young people hate to be different from their friends and classmates. So it's hard on an eight-year-old girl if she is the first in her class to begin developing breasts and shooting up in height, especially if she has doubts anyway about the pleasure of being an adult. (The girl who has always been wild to grow up may be happy to be an early developer.)

The early-developing girl has a special worry about how excessively tall she will end up in adulthood. She was probably one of the taller girls even before there was any prepuberty growth spurt. Then let's say she grew six inches in height between the ages of eight and ten years, while most of her classmates grew three. So at ten she towers above her classmates and worries whether she is going to end up a giantess who will scare all the boys away. Actually, from the time of her first period at ten, she will probably grow only two more inches altogether—so she is almost at her adult height now. And most of her classmates at age ten still have seven or eight more inches to grow, so they will do a lot of catching up.

At the other extreme, the girl of thirteen who hasn't begun her prepuberty growth spurt may be the shortest in her class as a result and the only girl who has not developed visible breasts. So she feels like a runt and wonders whether she will remain a child for life. She can be almost guaranteed that she will grow a total of seven or eight inches from the time her puberty growth spurt begins—and that is a lot of inches.

Though the average boy begins the puberty growth spurt at about twelve, there are quite a number who start as early as eleven or as late as thirteen, a few at ten or fourteen and an occasional one at nine or fifteen.

In our kind of society, where size and athletic ability are so important for boys, the early-developing boy who shoots up above his classmates is not so apt to be alarmed or displeased as the early-developing girl. But the boy who's on a slow schedule, who has probably always been on the small side of average anyway and who then is further left behind when most of his classmates get their growth spurt, is apt to assume he will be a dwarf and be deeply discouraged. But he can be assured that he will grow eight to ten inches from the time when his growth spurt begins—no matter how long he has to wait for it to start.

The External Genitals

The external genitals are those which can be seen; the internal genitals are inside the body.

In the boy the external genitals are the penis and behind it the scrotum, the sac which contains the two testicles.

The penis has a single tube inside, the urethra, through which passes the urine when the bladder is being emptied. And, during orgasm (which is the climax of sexual excitement), the semen, the fluid which contains the sperm, passes through it.

The penis is one or two inches long in childhood, but during puberty development it grows to three or four inches long and becomes considerably wider in diameter.

The penis has a head, or glans, which is marked off from the shaft by a groove (much like a neck). The skin of the shaft is thick and loose like the skin over the rest of the body. But the skin of the head of the penis is thin, tightly adherent to the underlying tissues, and highly sensitive; its colour, in a white person, is dusky bluish.

When a boy is born, the head of his penis is covered by a sleeve of skin called the foreskin. Later in childhood the foreskin becomes loose enough so that it can be pulled back over the head of the penis with ease, exposing it. (This would be like pulling an overly long sweater-sleeve up the arm, which eventually exposes the fist.) Various societies have designed ceremonies in which the foreskin is cut off ('circumcised', meaning cut around), leaving the head of the penis exposed. In the Jewish religion, circumcision is performed as a religious ceremony a few days after birth. The official purpose is cleanliness. In some 'primitive' societies circumcision is performed during adolescence, as part of the initiation of the youth into adulthood.

In present-day America, circumcision is very commonly performed shortly after birth mainly for reasons of cleanliness. The foreskin secretes a cheese-like material called smegma, which collects there between the foreskin and the head of the penis. It looks unclean, has an odour and sometimes becomes infected. Circumcision eliminates these problems. In Britain circumcision is far less common, mainly because people feel that the operation may inflict unnecessary pain. However, it may be necessary in some cases later on for medical reasons.

The penis is made of erectile tissue, meaning tissue largely composed of minute blood spaces. Ordinarily it hangs downward. When the spaces are tightly filled with blood, the penis becomes enlarged and stiff, and stands erect, somewhat the way a rubber balloon becomes enlarged and stiff when filled with compressed air. This engorgement of the penis with blood is brought about, anatomically speaking, by an increased arterial blood flow to the penis and a constriction of the veins through which the blood ordinarily leaves the penis. Psychologically speaking, the erection is caused by a sexually stimulating situation—physical contact with a girl (as in intense kissing, embracing, fondling), seeing a girl undressing, even thinking about an intimate situation with a girl. In this way the penis is prepared for insertion into a girl's or woman's vagina.

The testicles are two olive-shaped organs which lie in the scrotum, a pouch made of wrinkled brownish skin which hangs down behind the penis. The testicles manufacture the sperm which, when united with the ova (eggs) formed by females, develop into babies. (The word 'sperm' is both singular and plural. 'Ova' is the Latin plural for 'ovum'.) A testicle is composed of one long microscopic tube (like a ball of string), folded on itself countless times. It produces millions of sperm each week, from adolescence to old age.

As the sperm mature, they travel through the tube to small storage sacs called seminal vesicles located behind the prostate gland, which lies between the base of the penis and the rectum. (The doctor examines the prostate gland during a physical examination by putting his finger in the rectum and feeling in a forward direction.) In the seminal vesicles the sperm are mixed with semen, a thick fluid with a sticky consistency, a milky colour and an odour like that of sodium hydroxide. At the climax of a period of sexual excitement, orgasm occurs, during which the semen is ejected from the erect penis ('ejaculation') in a series of spasms, which produce a sensation of intense pleasure.

There is pubic hair on the scrotum and around the base of the penis but not on the penis.

In a girl the clitoris and the vagina are ordinarily closed in and concealed by folds of skin which run from front to back between the thighs. The outer folds are larger ('labia majora', meaning larger lips) and are covered with ordinary skin on the outside. After puberty this skin is wrinkled, brownish and covered with hair. When the outer folds are pulled aside there appear two smaller inner folds ('labia minora', small lips) which are of delicate moist skin (mucous membrane) somewhat similar to the lining of the mouth. At the forward end of the labia minora, partly visible between the labia majora, is the clitoris. It corresponds to the penis, in the embryological sense. (In the development of the embryo, both sexes start anatomically the same, but then certain organs are elaborately developed in one sex, inhibited in the other.) The clitoris is about the size of the lower edge of a girl's ear lobe, of firm, slightly erectile tissue, and very sensitive. Next behind the clitoris lies the opening of the urethra, for the passage of urine. Behind the urethra is the opening of the vagina, which leads to the uterus, or womb. ('*Vagina*' is Latin for 'sheath', since the vagina is thought of as a sheath for the man's penis). The vagina is an elastic structure that can easily be stretched. Partly covering the entrance to the vagina in the young girl is an extremely thin fold of rather insensitive skin called the hymen or maidenhead. It must be torn (the way a thin blister can be broken) before the penis can enter the vagina for the first time. The expressions 'lost her maidenhead' and 'lost her virginity' refer to the first time a girl has intercourse. If a girl has not lost her maidenhead before marriage, she may have a physician cut it before her wedding to be sure that there is not any pain to mar her wedding night.

The Internal Genitals

The uterus, or womb, is the organ designed to contain and nourish the baby while he grows from a microscopic embryo. The walls of the uterus are largely composed of muscle, for eventually expelling the baby. When not pregnant a uterus is the shape and size of a very small pear, with the large end up. It is nearer the size of a basketball at the time of birth. The narrow lower end of the uterus is called the cervix, which means the neck, and this contains the opening through which the sperm enters and the baby emerges. The vagina is attached to the uterus around the cervix.

From the sides of the upper, larger end of the uterus come two tubes (fallopian tubes, called tubes for short) which extend out towards the two ovaries. The ovaries, which are olive-sized, contain the eggs which mature, one every month, from the time a girl has her first period until the menopause (end of menstrual periods) at about the age of forty-five. The mature ovum breaks from the surface of the ovary (like a blister breaking), enters the open end of the fallopian tube and moves down it towards the uterus. If intercourse takes place about midway between menstrual periods (from eighteen to twelve days before the next period), one of the million sperm from the man's ejaculation, having swum into the cervix of the uterus, up through the central space in the uterus and out into one of the tubes, meets the ovum there, and penetrates its delicate exterior. The chromosomes (threadlike structures in the nucleus in the centre of egg and sperm), which carry the genes that will determine all the characteristics of the new individual, get together and the embryo starts to develop as it moves down the tube. By the time the fertilised egg enters the uterus it has formed minute tentacles with which it will attach itself to the lining of the uterus. These enlarge and multiply until they form a thick plaque, the placenta, which eventually becomes the size of a large Danish pastry and which is attached to the inside of the enlarged uterus. Between the placenta and the embryo's navel runs the umbilical cord. It contains the blood vessels through which the embryo gets the nutrients by which he will grow and through which are carried back to the placenta his waste materials. It is in the spongy spaces of the placenta that the exchanges of materials between the baby's blood and the mother's blood take place, across incredibly thin membranes. That is to say, the bloods of mother and embryo are not mixed.

When the nine months gestation (carrying or pregnancy) is completed (and nobody knows what signal is given) the uterine muscle starts to contract, first at long intervals. This is the beginning of labour. At some point in the process, the amniotic sac in which the baby has been suspended bursts and several pints of the watery fluid come out of the vagina. The baby, who is usually upside down in the amniotic fluid, with his head already 'engaged' (fitted) within the cavity of the mother's bony pelvis, is pushed downward by the pressure of the contractions of the uterus on his plump behind. His head pushing against the cervix slowly, over a period of hours, forces it open. The contractions gradually come more quickly, eventually five minutes apart, and the head is, little by little, pushed down the vagina. As it presses from the inside on the tissues around the opening of the vagina, it numbs them, so that the extreme stretching, which sometimes results in a tear of the skin, is not painful.

The contractions of the uterine muscle, after the cervix is opened, are of a quality which makes the mother push hard and this helps the baby along. The contractions have always been called labour pains and they are painful enough to make some women cry out. Others call their pains hardly noticeable. There are some doctors who believe that the fear of labour pain which has been instilled in women since the beginnings of recorded history (the Bible says that women must bring forth their children in pain as punishment because Eve ate the apple of knowledge) makes them react with a mental and bodily tension which causes most of the pain. These doctors teach pushing-down exercises and proper breathing throughout the pregnancy, so that women can co-operate with their uterine contractions in 'natural childbirth'.

Menstrual Periods

On the average of once every twenty-eight days, from puberty until about the age of forty-five, the lining tissue of a woman's uterus goes through a change which prepares it to receive and nourish a fertilised ovum. When no fertilised ovum appears, the material of the lining layer is shed, along with considerable blood-tinged fluid. This discharge lasts four or five days on the average. It is variously known as a period, a monthly, or 'the curse'. In earlier generations girls were brought up expecting to feel sick and weak during their periods, to have abdominal cramps, to be unable to participate in any vigorous physical activities. Gradually it was realised that most of these disabilities were induced in girls by the anxious overconcern of their mothers. Now we've swung so far in the opposite direction that the occasional girl who has sharp cramps is made to wonder whether she is imagining or exaggerating them. Girls who feel able to do so are now encouraged to keep up all their regular activities, including athletics, even swimming. Quite a few girls, though, feel irritable and slightly depressed.

Some girls have stopped wearing external pads (called by manufacturers 'sanitary towels') in favour of absorbent tampons, shaped like a fat cigarette, which can be worn inside the vagina and pulled out by the string which is attached to it.

In the first years of adolescence quite a few girls have periods which are not typical. They may come sooner or later than twenty-eight days or quite irregularly. Periods may be missed altogether, especially in summer, occasionally for a whole year after the first period. They may last a shorter or longer time than five days. There may be little discharge or an excessive amount. The cramps may be

147

severe. Almost none of these irregularities indicate abnormality or ill health. Almost all of them improve with time. It's good to consult a gynaecologist if there is no progress.

Nocturnal Emissions

By the time a boy is well into puberty development, he begins to have orgasms during dreams of sexual experiences in which there is ejaculation of semen. This is called a nocturnal emission or a wet dream. The boy finds the liquid on his pyjamas if the dream has been recent, or it may have dried into a crusty spot. The amount of fluid ejaculated is about one teaspoonful, though it seems more.

Any male who is not having intercourse regularly is bound to have nocturnal emissions and they have no other significance. They do not weaken the individual. The frequency is not important.

Contraception

There are a variety of ways to try to prevent the conception of a baby. One that has been used for centuries is for the man to withdraw his penis just before his orgasm occurs. This is quite unsatisfactory for both partners. A woman's orgasm usually doesn't come until the man's does so she is apt to be left dissatisfied by the man's withdrawal. The man may have his orgasm anyway, but it's very unnatural and unsatisfactory for him to pull away from the woman at this moment. And some of the semen may leave the penis before the full orgasm occurs.

A second method is for the couple to avoid intercourse during the days in the woman's menstrual cycle when fertilisation is likely to take place. This is called the Rhythm Method and is the one permitted by the Catholic Church because no artificial interference has been used. It requires intelligence on the part of the woman to keep track of the likely period, especially if her periods are at all irregular. It also requires self-control on the part of both husband and wife.

A method which has been used for many years is for the man to wear a thin rubber condom over his penis during the latter part of intercourse. This was considered a reasonably satisfactory method when there was nothing much better. The man has to be careful to put the condom on in time. (Since it has to be rolled on, as a stocking is sometimes rolled on to the leg, it can't be put on until there is an erection; so lovemaking has to be interrupted for a few seconds.) Some men dislike a condom because they think it interferes with their sensation, but most men would say this does not make a noticeable difference. A more serious fault for some men is that they lose their erection with any interruption of intercourse.

Considered better than the condom by most couples is the dome-shaped rubber diaphragm for the woman, filled with a jelly which kills sperm. The woman inserts it in her vagina in such a position that the dome and the jelly surround the cervix of the uterus, blocking the way for the sperm. When you see such a diaphragm it will look too large to fit in the vagina. But a vagina is very stretchable and the diaphragm, which can be squashed to about a quarter or less of its width to help insertion, has to be large enough so that the rim will stay wedged in the right position. The woman can put the diaphragm in position in advance of going to bed or at any other time when lovemaking is likely, and should leave it there at least eight hours, to kill any viable sperm. The diaphragm is prescribed and first

149

fitted by a physician. A person's own family doctor, or a doctor at one of the Family Planning Association's clinics, or Brooks' Advisory Clinics are the best people to give advice in confidence on all aspects of contraception.

The commonest failure of the diaphragm method occurs when the wife doesn't anticipate lovemaking, doesn't get the diaphragm in place in advance, and her husband is too impatient to wait for her to do it. Diaphragm and jelly are also fairly expensive.

More efficient and much less expensive is the so-called 'intra-uterine device', known as I.U.D., which has been used in recent years. This is a small coil of plastic which the physician places inside the uterus (through the cervix), where it is left in place for months at a time. A thread leading through the cervix into the vagina reassures the woman that the device is still in place. It probably works by preventing implantation of the egg in the womb.

The I.U.D. is being recommended all over the world where population is increasing too fast and where there is not enough money to supply the more expensive pill for the entire population. In Britain, however, it may not be recommended for use except by married women who have had at least one pregnancy.

'The pill' for contraception is composed of hormones which make the lining of the uterus resistant to the implanting of an ovum. It appeals aesthetically to women because they don't have to manipulate or investigate in the genital region and they don't have to interrupt lovemaking or plan ahead for it. Anxious men don't have to wonder about something being there which might interfere with their sensations or performance. But the pill is rather expensive for a majority of people and much too expensive for people in the non-industrialised parts of the world. It also requires the ability to follow directions about stopping the medication several days each month to allow menstruation to occur. Its regular use brings a very, very slight risk of abnormal blood clots in the veins, but most women are not deterred by this. There are greater risks in many of our actions . . . such as in crossing the street. However, smoking greatly increases the risk of thrombosis in association with the pill.

Abortion

In Britain the Abortion Act of 1967 states that if an unwanted pregnancy should occur, it may be medically terminated in a hospital under the National Health Service if two doctors agree that the continuance of the pregnancy would involve risk to the physical and mental health of the pregnant woman, or any existing children of her family, or if there is a substantial risk that if the child were born it would suffer from some serious physical or mental handicap. In reaching their opinion on the risk to the mother's physical or mental health, the doctors can take into account the conditions of her 'actual or reasonably foreseeable environment'.

[VI]
Physical Conditions

Venereal Diseases

There are a number of venereal diseases in America and Western Europe. Those which most people know about are called syphilis and gonorrhoea. Another of these diseases which has become increasingly common in Britain is known by the rather long name of non-specific urethritis. There are a few other rare venereal diseases and other minor conditions which can be caught by contact between the sexual organs, but which do not have effects on health nearly as serious as those resulting from syphilis and gonorrhoea.

In the old days a lot of people used to think that you caught V.D. just by having sexual intercourse with somebody to whom you were not married. Some people had superstitious ideas that marriage conferred immunity from venereal disease. Until the last few years it was in fact the case that venereal disease was unusual and caught mainly from prostitutes. But now, owing to the changes in sexual practices which have taken place recently, gonorrhoea at least is the second most common infectious disease in Britain, and a person is unlikely in fact to catch it from a prostitute, prostitutes being particularly well aware of how to avoid gonorrhoea.

Many young people are curious about how these diseases are caught and how they first originated. They are all infectious diseases caused by small organisms or germs of various kinds. You can catch a cold by breathing in the cold virus which has been sneezed or coughed into the air by somebody else. You may catch food-poisoning by eating food which somebody who has had food poisoning has handled, and whose hands have therefore contaminated the food with the germ. The germs causing venereal diseases are, however, much more delicate. They cannot survive outside the warmth and moisture of the human body. The idea of catching a venereal disease from a lavatory seat, therefore, is totally impossible. Young people often ask if you can catch V.D. by kissing. This can happen only under very rare circumstances. Normally you can only catch a venereal disease by its being passed from somebody who is already infected via the most intimate possible physical contact with another person. This means in the vast majority of cases by sexual intercourse. Anybody who has sexual intercourse with someone who already is infected with a venereal disease is extremely likely to catch the disease, for they are among the most highly infectious diseases in existence. If a person sleeps around obviously he or she has a greater chance of catching a venereal disease, but if they go steady, or wait to have intercourse until after marriage and marry somebody who has never previously had intercourse, then their chances of catching a venereal disease are slight. The point to be quite clear about is that today the young person who sleeps around has a good chance of catching a venereal disease, though it is unlikely to be syphilis.

People want to know how they can tell if they have a venereal disease. One of the problems associated with V.D. is that it is perfectly possible to have one of the diseases without knowing that you have got it, particularly if you are a girl. Syphilis and gonorrhoea produce different symptoms. Both, unlike many other infectious diseases, do not get better of their own accord. In fact, a venereal disease once caught is there for life unless it is treated.

A boy is quite likely to know if he has gonorrhoea. He will have a burning sensation as if passing boiling water when he urinates. He may have a discharge from the urethra which is coloured and smells unpleasant, particularly in the early morning. This is known as the gleet. Later he may have a generalised febrile, or feverish, illness rather like influenza. As the disease progresses the complicated tubes inside his body which serve the purpose of reproduction will become infected and he may become sterile and unable to father a child. Later he may find great difficulty in passing urine.

A girl is quite likely to have gonorrhoea without knowing that she is infected. If she does have symptoms she will have an offensive coloured discharge from the vagina, although of course some discharge is normal in adolescence and there are other causes of mildly infected discharges. In the later stages of the disease a girl may have fever and pain in the lower part of her stomach and it will be at this stage that her reproductive organs are being infected. As with the boy, she may end by becoming sterile and unable to bear children.

Syphilis is extremely rare in Britain, but its incidence has increased alarmingly over the last few years. Initially in either a boy or a girl the first sign is a shallow, pain-free ulcer on some part of the sexual organs. A boy, of course, will be able to see his ulcer, but in the case of a girl it could be inside the vagina or on the cervix and therefore invisible, and, as with gonorrhoea, she may not be aware of being infected. Later the ulcer will disappear and the person who does not know about the venereal diseases will feel a sense of relief and assume that the disease has cured itself. This is not, however, so. What has happened is that the germs have entered the body where the secondary stages of the disease are beginning to develop. This takes several weeks and may consist of a rash over the chest and back, and sometimes on the arms, and of a febrile illness and aches and pains. Some young people, knowing about this, have

confused the many kinds of rashes which teenagers sometimes get with syphilis and been badly and unnecessarily
frightened. Later, white ulcers, so-called snail-track ulcers,
develop in the mouth. These are filled with the germs of
syphilis and are highly infectious, and it is when somebody
has these ulcers that they can transmit syphilis by kissing.
This secondary stage of the disease will die down and again
the patient may assume that they are cured. However, years
—often ten or twenty years—later the third or tertiary stage
will develop when the syphilis germs will damage the heart,
the bones, the brain, and the blood vessels, causing death
due to insanity, or to rupture of a blood vessel or to heart
failure.

Non-specific urethritis is not nearly as alarming as either
syphilis or gonorrhoea but we do not yet know as much
about it as we should like to. Its initial symptoms both in a
girl and a boy are a discharge from the sexual parts and
local irritation.

Obviously if somebody thinks they have caught a venereal disease, and if they have taken the risk of sleeping with
somebody who is promiscuous they should bear this in
mind as a possibility, they will want to discuss the
matter in the greatest possible confidence. Almost all hos-
pitals in Britain have what are known as special clinics to
which anybody can go without a doctor's letter, and usually
without an appointment, and receive a test for V.D. and
suitable treatment. There is no need to go to the family
doctor and there is no need to fear that the matter will be
discussed with the patient's family. Anybody who goes to a
special clinic will, however, find that the social worker
there is anxious to discover where they caught the disease.
This is obviously sensible because the person who was the
source of infection is liable to infect other people. This
process, known as contact tracing, is handled with the

greatest delicacy and tact and only with the permission of the patient. It is very important for anybody going to a special clinic, however, to trust the discretion of the social worker and to co-operate in contact tracing.

The treatment of V.D. is simple and relatively painless, and usually consists of a series of injections of antibiotics.

All mothers are tested for V.D. early in pregnancy because doctors are aware that V.D. may affect babies. In the old days it was routine to treat babies' eyes at birth in case the mother had gonorrhoea, but this is only done today in Britain if it is known that the mother is infected.

Notices about special clinics for the treatment of venereal disease are often displayed in public lavatories, and most post offices display notices or will answer enquiries. It is natural for anyone to feel worried and ashamed about having to ask for directions, but so serious are these diseases that it is important to summon up the courage to do so.

Acne

In adolescence in both sexes the skin texture coarsens and the pores (hair follicles) enlarge, more so in boys. Adolescent skin becomes susceptible to acne—more in one individual, less in another. In acne the wax from the sebaceous (wax) glands, which are connected to the hair follicles (to keep the skin and hair oiled), collects in the follicles and hardens there. The top of each plug of wax, mixed with dirt, becomes a 'blackhead', which can be squeezed out with the fingernails, with some difficulty and pain. When the pores become plugged, it is easy for ordinary pus germs, which are usually on the skin anyway, to work down and cause infections under the plugs. These first show as red pimples, which later get white tops on them ('whiteheads') as the white blood cells collect to try to destroy the germs.

In spite of the fact that acne is so very common and causes so much mental anguish, very little that is useful is known about its cause or cure. It is not caused by sexual contact or by masturbation or by sexual thoughts, as some adolescents have guiltily imagined. You should consult a dermatologist if acne is troublesome.

Formerly a diet rich in sweets and chocolate was thought to be an important causative factor, but research has disproved that theory. The daily use of a soap containing hexachlorophene has been found helpful because it reduces the number of pus germs on the skin. Squeezing out the blackheads every month or so also helps. (Wash face and hands thoroughly with hexachlorophene soap first.) But don't squeeze a red (infected) pimple, or a whitehead, because the pressure tends to spread the germs through the surrounding tissues, which only makes a larger pimple and one which is therefore more apt to leave a scar. If an unsightly white top has formed, you can soften it by applying a piece of wet absorbent cotton for five or ten minutes and then try to wipe it off. (Also put a drop of hexachlorophene solution on the cotton to help prevent the spread of germs over the surrounding skin when the white top opens.) It's wise to try to keep your hands off your face if you have acne, because they spread the pus germs and rub them in.

Very helpful for improving the appearance of pimples is the use (by boys as well as girls) of a stick cosmetic which comes in various skin shades, in a case like a lipstick case. Pat the end of a finger on the tip of the cosmetic stick, then pat the finger on the pimple, aiming to get the heaviest concentration on the pimple itself, then shading off or blending the cosmetic into the surrounding skin. With practice you can make pimples almost unnoticeable, yet without giving an obviously made-up look. (Don't apply the stick directly to the pimple—the cosmetic is then too heavy and noticeable.)

When acne is very severe and leaves scars, a plastic surgeon sometimes recommends sanding off the outside skin under anaesthesia, which leaves—temporarily at least—a thinner, less easily infected skin. In a great majority of people, acne ceases to be troublesome in adulthood.

Body Odour

Body odours become much stronger in adolescence—partly as a result of glandular changes and skin changes, partly as the result of axillary (armpit) hair on which perspiration collects and is decomposed by bacterial action. It is essential that teenagers, in a society like ours which considers body smells offensive, take a careful soap or shower daily and follow with an underarm deodorant.

Hair and Scalp

Sweat is more profuse and oily in adolescence, which means that hair on the head gets to look greasy and straggly in a shorter time. Dandruff appears in winter and may become profuse. The hair should be washed once a week, more often if necessary. If dandruff is troublesome, a dermatologist should be consulted.

Most girls feel that the hair on their legs is dark enough so that they need to shave it once a week. (Shaving does not coarsen hair.) It can also be removed with a wax or chemical depilatory.

General Health Care

Many older adolescents and youths have an impulse to scorn health rules, to get along on little sleep, to eat a lopsided diet, as if proving their stamina and daring. To be sure, adolescence is a generally healthy age period. But occasionally there are physical diseases to which neglect contributes. It's worth keeping your body in good condition during this stressful period. Visit your doctor and dentist regularly. Eat a sensibly balanced diet.

In recent decades there has been a progressive increase in arteriosclerosis, including coronary heart disease, in young adults. It is suspected by some researchers, though not proved, that this is due to three factors. Most often blamed is a diet rich in animal fats, particularly the fat in meats, whole milk, butter; and also the cholesterol in eggs. A second suspected factor is cigarette smoking. A third is lack of exercise. Pending further knowledge it is not sensible to try to cut out all animal fats but only to cut off the extra fat from meat, to hold down on butter and cream, to drink mostly skimmed milk, to eat not more than two eggs a week.

[VII]
Smoking, Alcohol and Drugs

Tobacco

Having suffered miserably from the craving for cigarettes for three solid years after giving them up, and knowing the risk they entail for lung cancer and heart disease, I consider those people fortunate who have never become addicted. Their life expectancy is distinctly better. They'll never have the distress of withdrawal. They'll never miss the pleasure because smoking is not a pleasure until the taste is acquired.

Then why do people take up cigarettes? The main reason is the desire of young people to feel and appear grown up. The fact that throughout childhood parents have usually disapproved is an added inducement. I think that the danger of cancer and heart disease, far from discouraging the average young person, is a subtle challenge. It gives him another opportunity to prove to himself that he's willing to risk danger as unhesitatingly as the next man.

Certainly the desire to be grown up is one of the strongest motives in all human beings. Our species wouldn't get anywhere without it. But I'd strongly advise you to avoid cigarettes before you get hooked. Within a few years you'll feel grown up enough anyway (and soon begin to wish you were younger), so the habit will then have no useful purpose whatsoever. It will worry you for the rest of your life until you give it up.

You'd be impressed to see in a doctors' dining-room in a hospital how few doctors now smoke cigarettes. To them the danger is not a remote theory. They've seen too many people die of cigarettes to be able to enjoy them.

Pipes and cigars are much less harmful than cigarettes

but they appeal to relatively few people.

Smoking during pregnancy increases by thirty times the chances of death to the baby during labour or the first month of its life. Also the children of smoking mothers grow up to be slightly shorter in height, lighter in weight and of slightly less intelligence than those of non-smoking mothers.

Alcohol

Intoxicants are partly a matter of style. (Alcohol, marijuana and the addictive drugs are called intoxicants, meaning poisons, because they interfere with the normal functioning of the brain.) Alcoholic drinks (which are as old as civilisation) were used in unusually generous quantities by a large percentage of Americans between World Wars I and II. The Prohibition Amendment (which was ratified during the patriotic fervour of World War I) probably did a lot to make hard drinking more popular by making it illegal and thus more exciting. And it was considered dashing by a considerable proportion of students to drink heavily at weekends, especially on the occasion of games and dances. A few could always be counted on to vomit or pass out or both.

Heavy drinking was losing a lot of its popularity among students and others in the 1940s and 50s even before marijuana and other drugs gave alcohol competition.

Alcoholism is a disease, usually progressive, in which the person has an almost irresistible craving for drink, either in episodes or daily. In each episode he is incapable of stopping voluntarily, so he drinks to the point of incompetence. A great majority of alcoholics eventually lose their jobs because of failure to report for work or reporting drunk. The social disgrace of joblessness and of drunkenness at home and in the neighbourhood, and the tendency of many alcoholics to be abusive at home play havoc with family life. Alcoholics are usually contrite after an episode and full of promises which are never kept. The best record for cures is that of Alcoholics Anonymous, which provides sympathetic companionship, group discussion and a member to keep constant vigil with an individual who fears that an episode is coming on. But to be helped by A.A., an alcoholic has to be honest enough to admit that he is an alcoholic and needs help. Most alcoholics, though, won't admit they have the disease. They claim that they can stop drinking any time they wish, and go from bad to worse. The alcoholics in any country are roughly in proportion to the people who drink 'socially'. In other words, certain people with certain personality weaknesses are first introduced to social drinking and then go on to alcoholism. Most of them presumably would not have become alcoholics in a country in which social drinking was not popular.

The appeal of social drinking to most people is that it makes them feel less tense, less self-conscious, more self-assured, more sociable. They feel that they are more skilful in bodily co-ordination (in driving a car, for instance), more eloquent and witty in speech, more romantically seductive. But observation shows that performance in such spheres actually is impaired.

The moderate use of alcohol has been not only condoned but even recommended, for thousands of years, as an antidote to the strains of civilisation, and I don't deny its values and pleasures. Young people should recognise, however, that society's sanction does not mean that drinking is harmless; drinking takes a terrible toll among the millions who become alcoholics. It is also one of the major contributing causes of traffic deaths. This is especially true when the drivers are boys and young men who haven't had to face the fact yet that they are just as capable of bad driving-judgment as the next man, and who are eager to demonstrate that they have just as much rash courage as anyone.

Don't drive if you've been drinking and don't let anyone drive you who has been drinking. Better to be called chicken or square than to be dead or to cause the death of others.

I'd advise anyone who asked me that he should not drink at all until eighteen and preferably not until twenty.

Marijuana

Marijuana has become very popular in recent years among young people, although to be in possession of it, as with other drugs, is a criminal offence in the United Kingdom. This drug is not physically habit-forming (as morphine, cocaine, heroin are) but may be psychologically habit-forming. This means that the habitual user does not become physically sick and panicky when he cannot get the drug, the way users of morphine, cocaine and heroin do, but may become psychologically addicted in the sense of depending on it, feeling that he must have it, the way people become psychologically addicted also to ordinary sedatives like phenobarbitone or a stimulant like Dexedrine.

The users of this drug and most drug experts make the point that it is wrong to lump this drug with the physically addicting drugs and to punish those found in possession of it as harshly as if they possessed the addicting drugs. They also point out correctly that the fact that a certain number of people go from marijuana to more dangerous drugs doesn't prove that the marijuana led them to the other drug. I agree with these points, without being an expert in any sense. But I don't think that I or the experts have enough data yet to say marijuana is harmless. On this point, the experts disagree. The larger the number of people who use this drug, the larger the number who will become psychologically addicted. And I think it is sensible for me to assume, until proved wrong, that if a lot of people were accustomed to taking a mild drug, it will be easier for at least a few to go on to something more risky. To hear the protest that marijuana is no worse than alcohol, as so many users insist, doesn't reassure me. Alcohol becomes ruinous to an appreciable proportion of drinkers. I can accept the statement that most users of marijuana use it without apparent harm, like most users of alcohol. But I would still advise my teenage son or daughter not to become a user of either, during this difficult transitional period when so many aspects of personality are in an unstable state, when the die is being cast for decades to come, and when quite a few individuals get off the track anyway, psychiatrically, educationally or occupationally. I'd assume that by the age of twenty my son or daughter had as much stability as I and would have no need of my advice.

[VIII]
Delinquency

Conscience and Punishment

The first thing to realise about juvenile delinquency is that it's not one type of misbehaviour but an overall term for everything for which an adolescent may be haled into court, from parking offences to murder. It's as if everything that an adult could do wrong were called adult turpitude, a label which would certainly hinder rather than aid the understanding of different types of adult offences. The reason why all juvenile offences have been lumped together has been to get young people into special courts where, it was hoped, their difficulties could be understood and dealt with constructively rather than punitively; if they had to be removed temporarily from society, they would not be jailed with confirmed adult criminals but placed in rehabilitation institutions.

The question of conscience is important in any discussion of delinquency—the conscience of the individual, of the members of his family and of the social group to which the family belongs. The burglar or robber has a defective conscience. You can be sure that he was raised either by parents who had defective consciences too, or else by parents who didn't love him much; he may have resented this and never had the motive to try to live up to their standards. To put it positively, the reason most people behave well most of the time is that as young children they were warmed and comforted by their parents' love; they felt miserable when their parents temporarily disapproved of them; so they wanted, most of the time anyway, to retain that love by being good. Also they wanted very much to grow up to be like their parents and this meant doing things properly, too. People do not do the right things primarily because of fear of punishment. Punishment is only a vigorous reminder of disapproval. If the person being punished has never been loved enough to care whether he's approved of or not, the punishment does no good. This is shown by all the confirmed criminals who commit new crimes almost as soon as they get out of jail.

As you grow up you want to be approved of also by teachers, bosses, friends and society generally. Conscience is what tells you what your parents and society will and will not approve of.

The consciences of people in different social groups are not the same. Attitudes towards truancy are an example of this. In the family in which the parents left school as soon as they were able and see no great point in education, the average teenage son may not have much respect for schooling and may not be a particularly good student. Also, in such families the parents are apt to give up trying to control their children when they get beyond the stage when they can be punished physically. When a boy with no respect for education becomes physically full grown by fourteen or fifteen, he may have no patience with a female teacher who scolds him in front of others, and he may simply refuse to come back for more. His family may not try to persuade him to return, either. This contrasts with the family with high expectations where the parents control mainly by instilling in their children's consciences a strong sense of social and moral obligation which persists through adolescence and adulthood. They do this by frequently reminding their children of what is approved and disapproved—by society, by church, by family. They emphasise the long-term consequences of failure to live up to the expectation of their level of society; for example, that poor results in

171

school mean no further education, an inferior job, painful loss of respect from others and self.

To the boy brought up by parents who've always expected him to go to university, staying away from school would be a serious crime which he wouldn't dare commit unless he were intensely resentful about some injustice committed by the school authorities or unless he had been raised with a defective conscience.

In one social group, any stealing or cheating is looked on with horror. But in another it's not considered immoral to help yourself to some of the products of the factory, or goods at the shop, where you work. A majority of university students consider it all right to cheat an organisation (e.g., an insurance company) but not an individual. (This seems shocking as well as shortsighted to me.) In England they say you can leave a suitcase unattended indefinitely on a small-town railway-station platform, but in plenty of other countries it would be gone in ten minutes.

There are more offences committed *per capita* in late adolescence and early adulthood than at later age periods, for several reasons. Youths feel a rebellious rivalry with parents, teachers, police and other people in authority. They have a compulsion to prove their courage and independence. Their sexual and aggressive impulses are now fully grown but are not yet fully controlled by the caution that comes—fortunately or unfortunately, depending on how you look at it—with experience.

If we want to understand the various kinds of offences for which youths can be charged, we should separate them. First I'll mention mild delinquencies, of which a good example is petty larceny, which is snitching an apple from the stand in front of a fruit shop or a few pieces of timber at a building site. Studies have shown that four out of five respectable male citizens did such things at least once during adolescence, usually in a group, but that most of them had the good luck not to get caught. Such offences are motivated by the heightened masculine aggressiveness of adolescence (girls rarely commit them), or a need to prove one's boldness (a dare is often involved). Only a small proportion of boys are brought up strictly enough so that they wouldn't do any of these things.

A moderately serious offence would be a group of boys breaking into a school and deliberately destroying a lot of property. This is called vandalism. It requires considerably more hostility and aggression than most boys have, and less conscience. Incidentally, it also probably means that the school people as a group (or the particular teacher if only one room was vandalised) are hostile to the children of the neighbourhood. Another serious offence would be a group of boys from comfortable homes carrying out a series of burglaries of neighbourhood shops. In spite of the fact that the families are 'respectable' according to the newspapers, you can be sure that the parents have consciences less reliable than those of their neighbours or that they have neglected or mishandled their sons.

Armed robbery, which might end in shooting, and rape, both of which are very serious offences, are generally carried out only by boys who had been raised with little love and a lot of cruelty.

Girls tend to commit offences which are quite different from boys, and which show how different their basic natures are. They run away from home when they feel unappreciated and resentful, and this of course makes their parents frantic with worry and embarrassment. Usually in the background there is inadequate affection and a lot of family strain. The girls involved are often immature and self-centred.

Another common offence for girls is sexual delinquency.

A defiant girl may be keeping company with a man her parents consider no good, and her parents turn to the police and courts in their efforts to get her back under their control. There are other girls who scandalise their parents and the neighbours by appearing to be promiscuous with a variety of men. In these situations, too, there has often been too little love and too few standards.

So girls tend not to defy the law with aggression directed against society, like boys. They take a personal kind of revenge against their parents by worrying them and shaming them, often using their sexuality as the weapon.

Girls from mildly delinquent families may participate in shoplifting. In ordinary shoplifting, the objects stolen are of definite use or value to the person. But there is another variety called kleptomania in which a girl keeps taking more of the same object, which may have no practical usefulness at all. One favourite object of kleptomaniacs is pens—sometimes a girl will steal dozens and dozens of them. Some kleptomaniacs are financially well off and could easily buy the things they risk social disgrace by stealing. They have no idea why they keep stealing the same thing—it's a mysterious craving. But psychoanalysis has shown that in the unconscious the repeatedly stolen object has great symbolic significance.

[IX]
Relations with Parents

Gaining their Confidence

It's the nature of young people to be critical of their parents at times and to feel that most of the misunderstandings between them are the fault of the parents. (A critical attitude helps young people to leave home eventually.) They have always complained, with more or less justice, that parents are out of touch with modern ways, that they are possessive and bossy, that they lack confidence in their children's ability to cope with social and sexual crises; that they harp unnecessarily on certain issues, that they lack a sense of humour, at least in regard to parent–child relationships.

I think it's true that parents often underestimate their teenagers' capabilities and forget how they themselves felt in youth. When my future wife, Jane, and I told our parents in 1926—at the time I was in the middle of medical school with no prospect of earning a living for at least six more years—that we wanted to get married and that Jane would support us by getting some kind of job, though she had no training, they were dismayed. They said, 'But you can't live on an income like that!' We thought they were hopelessly timid and materialistic. In the end they gave in—against their better judgment. Thirty years later one of our sons, then finishing university and already married, said that he had decided to become a schoolteacher, though schoolteachers' salaries were miserably low at that time. Jane and I were taken by surprise. We exclaimed in dismay, 'But you can't live on an income like that!' He and his wife obviously thought that we were hopelessly timid and materialistic.

One reason parents are nervous about what their teenage children may do is that they still remember the troubles they themselves got into at that period and the more serious troubles that they almost got into—through inexperience, through wanting to carry off a situation rather than back out, through taking unnecessary chances. Over the years they've heard of the tragedies of youths in the families of acquaintances or fellow townspeople. Life has made them more pessimistic or at least apprehensive, whereas young people are almost invariably optimistic.

Young people like doing things on the spur of the moment and improvising. It's one of their ways of showing their ability to rise to a challenge and to make do. Older people startle easily; most of them plan things ahead, at least in the back of their minds, and are bothered by having their schedule interrupted by something quite unexpected. So when you want to borrow the family car or get your mother to do a sewing job, you'll have better success if you can possibly make your request in advance.

Youths make it harder for their parents to trust them because they can't resist the temptation to shock them. They say things like, 'Everybody we know drives at ninety miles an hour.' Or 'We've all decided we won't study for final examinations—it's useless.'

Young people often irritate their parents with their choices in clothes and hair styles, in entertainers and music. This is not their primary motive. They feel cut off from adulthood, into which they are not accepted yet. So they have to make the best of their separate status by having a society and culture of their own, to which they want to belong closely. Then if it turns out that their music or entertainers or vocabulary or clothes or hair styles irritate their parents, this is additionally enjoyable to youths because it suggests that they have the upper hand, at least in a

177

small way, and have seized the leadership in style and in taste.

Rebelliousness and pride can make you reluctant to curry favour with the parental generation—it seems like treachery to your own age group. However, this feeling is based on the assumption that you are the underdog, who cannot win but who can at least cling to his honour. This passive way of looking at things is natural enough after the long years of childhood during which you were completely under your parents' control. But it doesn't take account of the fact that you are now in actuality assuming an increasing responsibility for yourself. Even if your parents seem slow to recognise this, the reality is that you are out of their sight more and more of the time; school people and the other adults you deal with are granting you more authority to speak for yourself. So you are acquiring and exercising the status of an adult whether or not your parents will face this. (All parents are ready in some respects, unready in others.) You will impress them with your maturity and hasten their granting you greater independence to the extent that you can now act the part of the sensible, self-assured adult rather than the difficult or complaining child. If and when you are ready to make the switch, you have to stop thinking of co-operation as simply giving in to parental domination. That's the passive feeling of the young child. You have to shift to a positive attitude. Co-operation can be part of *your* master plan to be the person in charge of your life. You charm others—especially parents—into doing things your way. You impress others with your sense of responsibility, initiative, thoroughness, so that they will yield the authority to you that you want. Basically this is the philosophy on which even high officials of corporations operate. Every adult in the world (except for a few absolute dictators) has to get his own way by impressing and winning the co-operation of others.

A great majority of teenagers are highly responsible about school jobs, but fewer carry this over into home chores. They feel too much rebelliousness against parents to want to seem to comply totally on a home job. Just as important, parents are often less tactful than teachers in the way they assign a job or give reminders before reminders are really necessary. You can get a deserved reputation for responsibility by getting chores done before your parents have a chance to prod you.

Coming home at night at the time agreed on is another effective way to gain trust and reputation, particularly for a girl. If circumstances make this impossible, you can usually telephone. You may say that parents are silly to act as if coming home on time means you've been good, and that coming home late means you've been bad. That's true. But when parents see that you are responsible about one matter, it gives them confidence, rightly or wrongly, that you're responsible in other ways too.

Parents and other older people are more impressed by politeness in teenagers than you would imagine. Everybody likes being treated with consideration. But in addition, adults sense, at least unconsciously, that adolescents harbour considerable antagonism towards them (because of rivalry) and so are particularly delighted to be treated cordially instead.

Blaming Parents

When I was working years ago in an adolescent guidance clinic, two fifteen-year-old girls were brought to see me within a month of each other with problems that happened to be practically identical. The reason I bring up these cases now is not because I want to focus on the particular problem, which was quite serious (social withdrawal), but because of the marked contrast in both cases between the way the girl presented it and the way her parents did. The girl saw the situation as almost the opposite of the way it appeared to her parents. If there had been only one such case I would merely have been baffled, and would have called it a fluke. But when a similar case followed before I got the first out of my mind, I had to think more about it. I came to realise that the normal adolescent's need to view certain situations in a drastically different way from his parents explains many of the misunderstandings that occur in this age period; and it sheds light on some of the strains that most teenagers are going through.

In each case when I asked the girl herself what the difficulty was, she replied that her parents had lost confidence in her and wouldn't let her do things they had permitted before. For instance, she said, they no longer allowed her to attend the school football games or the Friday night dances. Later, when I asked the parents what they saw as the problem (while the girl was in the waiting room), they said they were worried because their daughter had withdrawn from her friends and from extracurricular activities. For instance, they said, she now refused to go to the football games or to the dances at the school. You can see why I was startled. The unusually drastic contrast between the points of view in these cases was due to the severity of the mental crises these particular girls were going through. But that is how many truths about the mental functioning of ordinary people have been discovered—through the exaggerated reactions of disturbed individuals. Normal young people of both sexes yearn to become more masterful and sophisticated in coping with life's social, romantic and sexual challenges. Boys, in addition, feel the compulsion to prove their manliness. All adolescents realise—at least unconsciously—that they still lack some of the skill or the nerve to attempt many of the acts, great and small, that they daydream about carrying off. But their pride and their striving to grow up make them hate to admit these lacks and hesitancies—even to themselves. Instinctively they look for excuses and scapegoats. Their parents have always been the ones who have kept them from doing many things—throughout childhood. So it comes naturally for them as teenagers to reproach their parents for not letting them do things which they themselves don't really feel up to doing anyway.

To an adolescent who is upset and withdrawn, like one of the fifteen-year-old girls mentioned, it is agony to be on public display—at a dance, for instance, or when walking in front of the grandstand at a game. So if an invitation comes from someone in the gang, an instantaneous, automatic answer that will save one from having to face one's own present sense of inadequacy would be, 'My parents won't let me go.'

A thirteen-year-old boy who is highly law-abiding might give the same answer to a new acquaintance who suggests they look for trouble on New Year's Eve. So might a sixteen-year-old girl invited to go somewhere with a crowd older and faster than she is used to. In such situations the young person may realise frankly that he himself does not feel up to accepting the invitation and he is glad to be able to give the excuse that his parents wouldn't let him accept. More often, though, he is consciously aware only of his strong desire to go along, to try the new adventure, to prove his courage or skill. He suppresses the self-doubts. Then, if his parents turn down his request, all he feels consciously is his resentment against them.

There is a third variation of this fear of inability to meet a challenge. A young person when he goes to his parent to ask permission to accept an unusual invitation may present it so that it sounds more risky than it really is, so that the parent will not even hesitate in saying no. 'On Saturday the crowd is going to a low dive in Milldale and they want me to go along. I think it's the place where that man was shot last year.'

Sex Education

The popular theory is that parents should go over the whole matter of sex with their children at the beginning of pre-puberty development and then have additional talks with them from time to time through adolescence. The father is supposed to be the adviser to his son, the mother to her daughter. Actually, in most cases this proves to be surprisingly difficult, especially between father and son. The father usually has to brace himself to introduce the subject; and when he begins, his son is immediately embarrassed and alarmed. This only shows again that sex is a highly complex matter full of taboos even in a supposedly enlightened era. I think it's fair to say that every teenager feels at least slight embarrassment or guilt about his own sexuality and is naturally reluctant to discuss the subject with his parents. The uneasiness dates back to when he was six or seven years old, but it is increased in adolescence because sex is so much more on his mind. And the fact that it was particularly towards the father that the boy felt guilty at six and seven explains why he still instinctively fears revealing anything of his sexual acts or thoughts to his father now.

A boy also doesn't want to have his father talk about sex

because it would remind him that his parents are still sexual beings, something he has wanted to forget ever since he suppressed his romantic attachment to his mother in early childhood. Most adolescents dislike and resist thinking of their parents as sexual beings.

I think discussion of sex with his son is difficult for a father because he too was brought up feeling guilty about the subject and he has an instinctive sense, despite modern progressive theories, that as a parent he should help to keep the subject repressed in the child for whom he's respon- sible. He can joke about sex (letting it out of repression) with a friend his own age because he has no sense of obliga- tion to teach morality to such a person, as he does with his son.

I have the impression from talking with many mothers that discussion of sex between them and their daughters is not as difficult as it is between fathers and sons, in a major- ity of cases. This is probably because most daughters are nowhere nearly as much in awe of their mothers as boys are of their fathers.

Mothers often end up talking with their sons about sex because their husbands never can get around to it.

I suspect that in Nature's scheme of things teenagers are expected to find out about sex by asking each other and their older brothers and sisters, and by keeping their ears and eyes open to remarks dropped by adults. Of course teenagers also turn to books, informative books directly focused on the facts of life, and novels and movies of the less inhibited kind. Many schools in Britain attempt sex education, phasing the programme to provide suitable in- formation at infant, junior, lower and upper secondary stages. In the final phase the teachers often call on outsiders to assist in group discussions with small groups of pupils. Young parents, family and school doctors, marriage guidance counsellors, trained by their national association, can all make valuable contributions.

I still think it's good for young people to hear about sex—not only the anatomical and physiological aspects, but the tender, spiritual and moral aspects, if this is possible—from the parents from whom they've learned so much else about life, so that it can all be fitted together in one integrated whole.

Parents don't teach about sex only on those rare occasions when they begin, 'There are some things that you and I need to talk about.' In ordinary dinner-table conversations there are bound to be discussions about such topics as what some of the wilder young people in the neighbourhood are up to and about the adult scandals of the town. Parents express their convictions in these discussions, and children listen without having to be told to.

The most important part of sex education, in the broad and true sense, is the example the parents set for their children. I mean the respect and tenderness they show for each other (even though they may have quarrels), the selfless co-operation in the care of the family, the mutual loyalty. If children have this kind of image of married love before them, they are getting a good basic education. The fact that such parents may possibly be too shy to discuss the anatomy and the intense feelings involved in sexuality is not so important. The missing pieces can be found elsewhere and fitted into the broad picture later.

[X]
Afterword

The Future

There are quite a few young people who have become disgusted with so many aspects of modern life in America and in Western society generally that they have turned their backs on the whole system: the readiness of leaders to make war on the flimsiest of rationalisations, barbaric racial injustice, the tolerance of poverty, second-rate education, inadequate medical care in the world's richest nation, the frantic competition for success, the focus on material possessions, the pollution of the environment, the exploitation of sex, to mention the worst.

Some youths have declined to take ordinary commercial jobs, or to live in overstuffed comfort, or to wear the conventional style of clothes. Some of them have gone to work as community organisers (on bare subsistence allowances) to try to help disadvantaged people to find ways to help themselves. Some have joined the Peace Corps in the same spirit. Such jobs combine idealism and realism.

A small number have even withdrawn into separate communities in which they share whatever food and other necessities are available and deliberately do without the comforts and luxuries, much as the early Christians did. Such an abnegation of the world can be a valuable preliminary step to the formulation of a new philosophy or religion.

Some young people, searching for an alternative to materialism, but unenthusiastic about Christianity and Judaism because these are their parents' religions and because they have not brought salvation (one trouble is that they

186

have never really been tried), want to hear about such religions as Buddhism and Hinduism, with their emphasis on contemplation and the quest for inner serenity. I do not know enough about them to estimate how much appeal they could have for Western society. I have a bias, because of my background and profession, in favour of man's trying to understand his own nature critically as a first step in getting out of all his present troubles, rather than of his cultivating a mystical otherworldliness. Then he can more wisely work for his family and humanity, which is what I believe he is designed for.

I think that man is naturally idealistic as much as he is naturally materialistic. Perhaps the main reason that young people are now showing idealism in wanting to work for humanity is that for the last twenty years so many in the older generations appear to have been exclusively interested in possessions.

I cannot produce a new religion for those who find the traditional ones uninspiring or unbelievable. But I do believe that man has great inner resources for creativity, dedication, love, generosity, enjoyment of arts and recreations. He is happier when he belongs to a group or society, when he feels that their welfare or their common ideal is a lot more important than his individual wants and when he works for their benefit. All this is not to deny that man is also capable of greed, power-seeking and cruelty. But the fact that man has these dangerous tendencies should not, I feel, make us hopeless or cynical. It should spur us on to find ways, through changing our educational methods, our commercial and professional aims, our governmental policies, to bring out man's better side. I mean his loving, serving, creative aspects. These are what have produced what civilisation we have. They could make a truly good world if we would put our technical knowledge and our material means at their disposal. The great and only hope for the future, as I see it, is that young people have glimpsed this vision and that they have the idealism and courage to work for it.

Suggested Books for Further Reading

K. C. Barnes, *He and She* Harmondsworth, Penguin Books, 1960

J. Dawkins, *A Textbook of Sex Education* Oxford, Blackwell, 1967
Young People and Sex London, S.C.M. Press, 1967

R. Dubos, *Mirage of Health* London, Allen and Unwin, 1960

J. Hemming, *The Problems of Adolescent Girls* London, Heinemann, 1967

Sir J. Huxley, *The Humanist Frame* London, Allen and Unwin, 1961

H.M.S.O., *Pamphlet 49. Health in Education*
Handbook of Health Education

M. O. Lerrigo, *Sex Education Series* London, Heinemann Medical Books

D. Morris, *The Naked Ape* London, Corgi, 1969

A. Myrdal and V. Klein, *Women's Two Roles* London, Routledge & Kegan Paul, 1968

D. Odlum, *Journey Through Adolescence* Harmondsworth, Penguin Books, 1960

Royal College of Physicians Reports, *Smoking and Health* London, Pitman, 1970

Sir Charles Sherrington, *Man on His Nature* Cambridge, Cambridge University Press, 1951

G. D. Shultz, *It's Time You Knew* London, Darwen Finlayson, 1968

P. T. de Chardin, *The Phenomenon of Man* London, Fontana, 1965

Index

Abortion, 151
Acne, 158–60
Aggression, 56–60, 63–4, 122, 126, 172–4
Alcohol, 165–8
Alcoholics Anonymous, 166
Animals, sexual relations in, 14, 24

Body Odour, 161
Breasts, 22, 53, 86, 138–9
Brooks' Advisory Clinics, 150

Childbirth, 145–6
Child-rearing, occupation of, 61–2, 66–70
Circumcision, 141–2
Climax, see Orgasm
Clitoris, 143–4
Cocaine, 167
  see also Drug addiction
Companionate marriage, 92
Condom, rubber, 149
  see also Contraceptives
Conscience, 170–1
Contraceptives, 30, 78–9, 131, 148–51
  see also separate entries for Pill, etc.

Dandruff, 161
Dating, 23, 58, 72–3, 76–8, 81, 83–4, 86, 90, 95–6, 106, 131
Daydreams, 12, 20, 24, 28, 31, 58, 125, 181
  see also Fantasies
Delinquency, juvenile, 170–4
  sexual, 178
Deviations, sexual, 116–27
Dexedrine, 167

Diaphragm, rubber, 149–50
  see also Contraceptives
Diet, 162
Divorce, 26, 49, 92, 122
Drinking, 165–8
  and driving, 166–7
Drug addiction, 47, 122, 125, 165, 167–8
  see also separate entries for Marijuana, etc.

Education, 40–2, 44, 131–2
  and sexual behaviour, 33–4, 37, 52
  and delinquency, 171–2
Erection, 132–4, 142
Ejaculation (emission), see Semen
Embryo, 144–5
Exhibitionism, 105–6

Falling out of love, 94–7
Fallopian tube, 144–5
Family Planning Association, 150
Fantasies, sexual, 30, 125, 131–2
  see also Daydreams
Fatherhood, 70
Freud, Sigmund, 13, 19
Frigidity, 135

Genitals, 16–17, 19–20, 28, 53, 86, 105, 131
  external, 141–4
  internal, 144–5
Gestation, see Pregnancy
Glands, sex, 12, 22–3, 25, 73–5
Gonorrhoea, 154–6, 158
  see also Venereal disease
Groin, ache in the, 132–3
Group companionship, 87–9

Guilt about sexuality, 29, 130–2, 183

Heroin, 167
  see also Drug addiction
Hexachlorophene, remedy against acne, 159
Hippie life, 46
Homosexuality, 117–21, 126
  and the law, 120
Hymen (maidenhead), 144

Identity, sense of, 43, 45–6, 130
Illegitimate child, 30, 98
  see also Pregnancy, illegitimate
Impotence, 55, 130, 133–4
Incest taboo, 28
Infertility, 133
Inhibition, sexual, 23, 30, 33–4, 52–3, 58–9, 84, 113, 123–4, 131–2
Intercourse, 52–5, 133, 142, 144–5, 148, 154–5
  before marriage, 31–2, 37, 74, 78, 131
Intra-uterine device (I.U.D.), 150
  see also Contraceptives

Jealousy, 19, 24, 94, 98, 115–16

Kinsey Reports, 32–4, 52–3, 118, 132
Kleptomania, 174

Labour pains, 146
Lechery, 114
Love, romantic, 17–19, 23–4, 26, 72–5, 77–8, 110, 114
  sexual-romantic, 26, 110
  possessive, 110, 115
  varieties of, 110–11
  see also Physical sex and love
Lovemaking, 35–6, 38, 56
  patterns of, 52–5
  see also Intercourse

Maidenhead, *see* Hymen

Marijuana, 165, 167–8
  see also Drug addiction
Marriage, 78 80, 98, 122, 131–2, 134, 154
  child's image of, 26–7, 48, 184
  intercourse before, 31–2, 37, 74, 78, 131
  meaning of, 47–51
  teenage, 51
  across barriers, 112–13
Masculinity, 15–16, 65, 120
Masochism, 121–3
Masturbation, 19, 28, 130–2, 159
Menopause, 66, 145
Menstrual periods, 138, 145, 147–8
Morphine, 167
  see also Drug addiction
Motherhood, 69
  see also Child-rearing
Non-specific urethritis, 154, 157
  see also Venereal disease
Nudity, 29, 105–7
Nursery schools, 66–70
Nymphomania, 125

Obscenity, 125–7
Orgasm, 53–4, 141, 142–4, 148
Ovaries, 22, 145
Ovum (egg), 142–3, 145, 147

Parents, *see* Relations with parents
Penis, 16–17, 19, 53, 60, 119, 132–3, 139, 141–3, 148–9
Petting, 85–6, 132
Phenobarbitone, 167
Physical attraction, 74–5, 113
Physical sex and love, 26, 72–6, 110, 114
Pill, the, 30, 78, 150–1
  see also Contraceptives
Pimples, *see* Acne
Popularity, 100–3
Pornography, 125–7
Possessiveness, 110, 115–16
Potency, 54, 57, 134
  see also Impotence
Pregnancy, 144–6, 158, 165
  illegitimate, 30, 78–9, 131

INDEX

Promiscuity, 73, 174

Prostitutes, 125, 154

Puberty, 22, 118, 138–40, 143, 147–8

Pubic (genital) hair, 22, 138–9, 143

Quarrels, 96–7, 122

Relations with parents, 14–22, 25–6, 39–41, 45–6, 63, 68, 79, 107, 110, 115, 170–4, 176–84

Rebelliousness, 39–43, 107, 172, 178–9

Religion, 186–7
and sexuality, 12–13, 28

Rhythm method, 149
see also Contraceptives

Rivalry with parents, 19–20, 39–41, 172
between the sexes, 60–5
with sister, 111

Romantic love, 17–19, 23–4, 26, 77–8, 110, 114
and physical sex, 26, 72–5, 110, 114

Sadism, 121–3

Scrotum, 141–2

Semen, 133, 141, 143, 148

Sex characteristics, secondary, 22

Sex criminals, 124–5

Sexual deviations, *see* Deviations

Sex Education, 182–4

Sexual fantasies, *see* Fantasies

Sex glands, *see* Glands

Sexual freedom, 30–3, 37, 64, 92

Sexuality, attitudes towards, 12–13, 27–8, 126, 132, 134
and religion, 12–13, 28
in childhood and adolescence, 13, 16–20, 22–7, 58, 82
inhibitions about, 23, 30, 33–4, 52–3, 58–9, 84, 113, 123–4, 131–2
guilt about, 29, 130–2, 183
and marriage, 47–8, 112

Shame about sex, 29

Shoplifting, 174

Shyness, 23, 58, 90, 99, 104

Smoking, 164–5

Sublimation of sex, 19, 21, 35, 52, 58

Syphilis, 154–7
see also Venereal disease

Teenage marriages, 51

Testicles, 22, 132–3, 139, 141, 143

Trial marriage, 92–3

Umbilical cord, 145

Uterus, 65, 144–5, 149

Vagina, 53, 133, 142–4, 146–7, 150, 156

Vandalism, 173

Varicocele, *see* Groin

Venereal disease (V.D.), 154–8
see also separate entries for Gonorrhoea, *etc.*

Virility, 56–7, 82, 134

Voice change, 22, 139

Womb, *see* Uterus